SITE-SPECIFIC CANCER SERIES

Head and Neck Cancer

Edited by
Linda K. Clarke, MS, RN, CORLN, and Mary Jo Dropkin, PhD, RN

Oncology Nursing Society
Pittsburgh, Pennsylvania

ONS Publishing Division
Publisher: Leonard Mafrica, MBA, CAE
Director, Commercial Publishing/Technical Publications Editor: Barbara Sigler, RN, MNEd
Production Manager: Lisa M. George, BA
Staff Editor: Lori Wilson, BA
Copy Editor: Amy Nicoletti, BA
Graphic Designer: Dany Sjoen

Site-Specific Cancer Series: Head and Neck Cancer

Library of Congress Control Number: 2005931424

ISBN 1-890504-55-6

Publisher's Note
This book is published by the Oncology Nursing Society (ONS). ONS neither represents nor guarantees that the practices described herein will, if followed, ensure safe and effective patient care. The recommendations contained in this book reflect ONS's judgment regarding the state of general knowledge and practice in the field as of the date of publication. The recommendations may not be appropriate for use in all circumstances. Those who use this book should make their own determinations regarding specific safe and appropriate patient-care practices, taking into account the personnel, equipment, and practices available at the hospital or other facility at which they are located. The editors and publisher cannot be held responsible for any liability incurred as a consequence from the use or application of any of the contents of this book. Figures and tables are used as examples only. They are not meant to be all-inclusive, nor do they represent endorsement of any particular institution by ONS. Mention of specific products and opinions related to those products do not indicate or imply endorsement by ONS.

ONS publications are originally published in English. Permission has been granted by the ONS Board of Directors for foreign translation. (Individual tables and figures that are reprinted or adapted require additional permission from the original source.) However, because translations from English may not always be accurate or precise, ONS disclaims any responsibility for inaccuracies in words or meaning that may occur as a result of the translation. Readers relying on precise information should check the original English version.

Printed in the United States of America

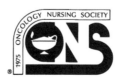

Oncology Nursing Society
Integrity • Innovation • Stewardship • Advocacy • Excellence • Inclusiveness

Contributors

Editors

Linda K. Clarke, MS, RN, CORLN
Formerly Head and Neck Nurse Specialist at the Milton J.
    Dance, Jr. Head and Neck Rehabilitation Center
Greater Baltimore Medical Center
Baltimore, Maryland

Mary Jo Dropkin, PhD, RN
Associate Professor
Long Island University School of Nursing
Brooklyn, New York

Authors

Lisa L. Blevins, RN, BSN, OCN®
Clinical Partner, Department of Radiation Oncology
Greater Baltimore Medical Center
Baltimore, Maryland
Chapter 7. Radiation Treatment and Symptom Management

Linda K. Clarke, MS, RN, CORLN
Formerly Head and Neck Nurse Specialist at the Milton J.
    Dance, Jr. Head and Neck Rehabilitation Center
Greater Baltimore Medical Center
Baltimore, Maryland
Chapter 1. Introduction

Margaret L. Colwill, RN, BSN, CORLN
Nurse Clinician, Head and Neck Oncology
Department of Otolaryngology
University of Iowa Hospitals and Clinics
Iowa City, Iowa
Chapter 4. Prevention and Early Detection

Cindy J. Dawson, RN, BSN, CORLN
Nurse Manager, Otolaryngology—Head and Neck Surgery
    Clinic, Oral Surgery Clinic
University of Iowa Hospitals and Clinics
Iowa City, Iowa
Chapter 5. Patient Assessment

Mary Jo Dropkin, PhD, RN
Associate Professor
Long Island University School of Nursing
Brooklyn, New York
*Chapter 1. Introduction; Chapter 8. Chemotherapy; Chapter
    11. Nursing Research Issues*

Penelope Stevens Fisher, MS, RN, CORLN
Clinical Instructor of Otolaryngology
Advanced Practice Nurse
Department of Otolaryngology: Head and Neck Service
University of Miami
Miami, Florida
Chapter 10. Survivorship

Margaret M. Hickey, RN, MSN, MS, OCN®, CORLN
Field Associate Director, Clinical Affairs
Tibotec Therapeutics
Bridgewater, New Jersey
Chapter 3. Pathophysiology

Helen Lazio-Stegall, RN, BSN, CORLN
Assistant Nurse Manager
Department of Otolaryngology-
Head and Neck Surgery
Department of Hospital Dentistry
Oral and Maxillofacial Surgery
University of Iowa Hospitals and Clinics
Iowa City, Iowa
Chapter 4. Prevention and Early Detection

Joan Such Lockhart, PhD, RN, CORLN, AOCN®, FAAN
Professor and Associate Dean for Academic Affairs
Duquesne University School of Nursing
Pittsburgh, Pennsylvania
Chapter 2. Anatomy and Physiology

Lenore K. Resick, MSN, CRNP, BC, NP-C, Doctoral
    Candidate
Associate Professor and Director
Nurse Managed Wellness Centers
Interim Director
Family Nurse Practitioner Clinical Specialty, Graduate
    Program
Duquesne University School of Nursing
Pittsburgh, Pennsylvania
Chapter 2. Anatomy and Physiology

Raymond Scarpa, MA, CNS, AOCN®
Advanced Practice Nurse
Department of Surgery, Division of Otolaryngology
University of Medicine and Dentistry of New Jersey
Newark, New Jersey
*Chapter 6. Surgical Management of Head and Neck Malig-
    nancies*

Ann E.F. Sievers, RN, MA, CORLN
Ear, Nose, and Throat Nurse Expert
University of California Davis Medical Center
Sacramento, California
*Chapter 9. Postoperative Management of the Head and Neck
    Surgical Patient*

Jill Solan, RN, MS, ANP, OCN®
Clinical Nurse
Memorial Sloan-Kettering Cancer Center
New York, New York
Chapter 8. Chemotherapy

Jose Zevallos, BA
Medical Student
University of Medicine and Dentistry of New Jersey
Newark, New Jersey
*Chapter 6. Surgical Management of Head and Neck Malig-
    ancies*

Contents

Foreword

This comprehensive resource for nurses and other healthcare professionals is the first of its kind—a classic text on the care of patients with head and neck cancer. It is a vital sourcebook for practitioners who are faced daily with patient care issues that have a significant impact on the quality of life following treatment for head and neck cancer. Therefore, it is with a sense of honor that I offer some introductory words to this excellent and long-awaited text.

It has been a pleasure to have known the editors for many years. Both are expert head and neck nurses and are particularly knowledgeable about the rehabilitation of this special population, having had extensive experience in the field for more than 35 years. While practicing at the Milton J. Dance, Jr. Head and Neck Rehabilitation Center in Baltimore, Maryland, Linda Clarke set an unparalleled standard of excellence for innovative head and neck cancer care. Mary Jo Dropkin, always on the forefront of self-care research, is well known for her valuable contributions concerning coping with disfigurement and dysfunction following head and neck surgery. Both have become nationally recognized experts in the management of head and neck cancer.

Linda and Mary Jo's mutual practice interest spawned a desire to work together in planning and producing this authoritative text. As expert and seasoned otorhinolaryngology and head-neck nurses, they had ready access to sources of new knowledge in the field of head and neck cancer nursing. Both have been long-time members of the Society of Otorhinolaryngology and Head-Neck Nurses and the Oncology Nursing Society and could draw upon the expertise of colleagues as well.

The editors selected an impressive team of authors from around the country to provide the reader with a sound understanding of head and neck cancer care. These clinical experts have contributed to the content of this informative book addressing contemporary care issues, both clinically and theoretically based.

Exciting times lie ahead for the management of head and neck cancer as new treatment options become available and nursing research seeks to answer and define important care questions. This unique book offers the practitioner a sound knowledge base using "state of the art" information in the approach to providing nursing care. Consider keeping a copy of this text at each practice setting so that you and others will have ready access to this valuable reference tool.

It is a privilege to present this book to its many potential readers.

Sandra L. Schwartz, MS, RN, CORLN
Executive Director
Society of Otorhinolaryngology and Head-Neck Nurses

Preface

The incentive for this book was driven primarily by the need for a comprehensive resource to guide staff nurses as well as advanced practice nurses in the delivery of safe and appropriate care to patients with head and neck cancer and their families. Although relatively uncommon, head and neck cancer is a devastating and complex illness that often results in permanent facial disfigurement and dysfunction. The disease process and treatment sequelae are accompanied by a myriad of physical, emotional, and social needs posing challenges to patients, families, and healthcare providers. Nurses play a crucial role in working collaboratively with all members of the healthcare team to coordinate and facilitate patient care across the continuum. We are heartened that advances in standard treatment modalities, including surgical approaches, radiation oncology, and medical oncology, as well as symptom management, are producing increased longevity and improved quality of life. However, the increasing number of survivors will need increased nursing awareness of their disease and treatment as well as compassion for the rigorous ordeal they may have endured. Caring for patients with head and neck cancer is one of the most demanding career paths a nurse can choose. It also is one of the most meaningful and most rewarding. This book, therefore, serves not only as a valuable resource on nursing care for patients with head and neck cancer but also as an introduction to the patients themselves—their courage, their spirit, and their will to survive despite enormous and unique adversity.

Acknowledgments

To the patients, physicians, and nurses who have taught and inspired me, to my late parents, Anna and Ernest Knoche, who encouraged me to become a nurse, and to my husband, Robert C. Clarke, whose love and support enabled me to pursue and achieve my professional goals.

Linda K. Clarke

Dedicated to the many patients with head and neck cancer for whom I cared and from whom I acquired the knowledge that now enriches my teaching.

Mary Jo Dropkin

CHAPTER 1

Introduction

Mary Jo Dropkin, PhD, RN, and
Linda K. Clarke, MS, RN, CORLN

Overview and Definition

Head and neck cancer often is considered to be the most devastating and debilitating of all cancers. Although other patient populations sustain similar morbidity with cancer treatment, the unique physiologic and psychosocial needs of patients with head and neck cancer emerge and are magnified by the facial disfigurement and multiple sensorimotor functional impairments associated with surgery, radiation therapy, and chemotherapy.

Many carcinomas of the oral cavity and pharynx are suited to early diagnosis because the involved sites are easily accessible to physical examination. Other cancers, however, originate in more "occult" sites and are less readily detected. The oral cavity includes the lips, buccal mucosa, lower and upper alveolar ridges, retromolar gingiva, floor of the mouth, hard and soft palates, and anterior two-thirds of the tongue. Pharyngeal structures include the nasopharynx, oropharynx, and hypopharynx. The nasopharynx, or superior portion of the pharynx, lies behind the nasal cavities and extends from the posterior nares to the level of the uvula. The oropharynx lies behind the oral cavity and extends from the uvula to the epiglottis. Within the oropharynx lie the faucial arches and palatine and lingual tonsils. The hypopharynx extends from the epiglottis to the openings of the larynx and the esophagus and includes the pyriform sinuses and base of the tongue (Montgomery, Lazor, & Weber, 2002). The primary site of head and neck cancer has a direct effect on the treatment plan and subsequent sequelae. For example, ablative surgery on the anterior tongue frequently results in permanent speech impairment; surgery involving the retromolar gingiva may result in a long-term swallowing deficit.

The American Cancer Society estimated that 67,060 new cases of head and neck cancer will occur in the United States in 2005, accounting for 12,810 deaths (Jemal et al., 2005). Although the overall occurrence of head and neck cancer represents only 5% of all newly diagnosed cancers, recent national statistics indicate that oral cavity cancer ranks in the top 10 leading sites of projected new cases in men; similarly, thyroid cancer ranks in the top 10 sites of projected new cases in women (Jemal et al.). Of 11 racial and ethnic groups investigated by the Department of Epidemiology and Surveillance at the American Cancer Society (1996), African American men have the highest rate of oral cavity and pharynx cancer (OCPC) at 20.4 per 100,000. More recently, distribution of cases by race and stage indicates that 37% of OCPC cases in Whites are diagnosed in the early stages (stage I/II) and another 57% in stages III/IV. Only 69% of OCPC cases are diagnosed early in African Americans, and 73% are not diagnosed until stages III/IV(Jemal et al.). Overall, five-year survival rates are 60% for Whites and 36% for African Americans. This represents almost a 50% increase in mortality rate for oral cavity cancers in African American males (Jemal et al.). Survival rates for larynx cancer are more equivalent, with a 67% five-year survival rate for Whites and a 51% survival rate for African Americans (Jemal et al.). Specific reasons for the disparity in these mortality rates by primary site and race remain unclear.

Vital Statistics

Cancers of the head and neck originate in the epithelial tissue. Squamous cell carcinoma accounts for 90%–95% of all head and neck cancers. The remaining 5%–10% are primarily adenocarcinomas of minor salivary gland origin or lymphomas, arising in the rich lymphatic network of this region (Harris, 2000).

Head and Neck Cancer and Substance Abuse

Risk factors for head and neck cancers include alcohol abuse and the use of all forms of tobacco (e.g., cigarettes, cigars, pipes, chewing tobacco). Approximately 75% of patients with oral cavity cancer are smokers (Scully & Porter, 2000). Active smokers also have a significantly higher rate of smoking-related second primary tumors of the oral cavity and pharynx (Khuri et al., 2001). Smokers who abuse alcohol as well have a 38 times greater risk of developing OCPC than nonsmokers/nondrinkers (Blot, 1992; Patten, Martin, & Owen, 1996). Risk factors that involve lifestyle are particularly relevant to recovery because of the high incidence of recidivism in smoking and alcohol consumption (Rose & Yates, 2001; Scully & Porter) and the development of local recurrence or second primary tumors as a result (Khuri et al.).

Other Risk Factors

The incidence of tongue cancer in adults younger than 40 who have no apparent risk factors is on the rise (Friedlander, Schantz, Shaha, Yu, & Shah, 1998). Overall, poverty and race continue to be risk factors, particularly in African Americans, who present with more severe disease and subsequently survive for a shorter period of time than Whites (Mood, 1997). Economic and social barriers to accessing medical treatment, however, confound this issue (Guidry et al., 1996). Other barriers to early cancer detection in minority populations include lack of knowledge about the increased risk of developing cancer, reluctance to undergo diagnostic procedures, and personal misconceptions about cancer diagnosis and treatment (Barroso et al., 2000; Foxall, Barron, & Houfek, 2001; Phillips, Cohen, & Moses, 1999; Robinson, Kimmel, & Yasko, 1995).

The U.S. surgeon general recently reported that, among all of the minority groups in the United States, cigarette smoking rates continue to be highest in African Americans (U.S. Department of Health and Human Services, 2000), clearly designating this group at extremely high risk for OCPC. Finally, some evidence is beginning to emerge suggesting that molecular changes in oral cancer may reflect not only etiology, such as tobacco and alcohol use, but ethnicity as well (Paterson, Eveson, & Prime, 1996). However, this has not been specifically documented, to date, in the U.S. population.

Head and Neck Cancer and the Older Adult

In the United States, older adults represent the most rapidly growing segment of the population. With advanced age comes an increased incidence of malignancies and comorbidities. Many factors related to carcinogenesis contribute to the development of cancer with increasing age. These include length of carcinogen exposure, decreased ability to repair DNA, loss of tumor suppressor genes, and decreased immune surveillance (Dessner, 2000).

In the general population, age is positively correlated with more advanced cancer at diagnosis with subsequent decrease in local control and disease-related survival (Allison, Franco, Black, & Feine, 1998; Clayman, Eicher, Sicard, Razmpa, & Goepfert, 1998; Jones, Beasley, Houghton, & Husband, 1998). Comorbidity and the tendency to attribute symptoms to the aging process frequently are reasons why the elderly fail to seek medical attention until the disease is in the advanced stages. Comorbidity, in turn, may preclude curative treatment, further contributing to poor prognosis (Hirano & Mori, 1998; Singh et al., 1998).

More than half of all patients with head and neck cancer are older than 65 years of age (Dropkin, 1999). Older adults also are more likely to be diagnosed with head and neck cancer at later stages because of the presence of physiologic changes occurring with aging that may mask the symptoms, particularly of oral cancer. These patients often are homebound and edentulous and, therefore, tend to visit the dentist infrequently. Thus, they should be targeted for early detection and screening programs (Aubertin, 1997).

Concerns often are raised regarding the efficacy of treatment in older patients with head and neck cancer, particularly when anesthesia and lengthy surgical procedures are being considered. However, recent research findings have revealed that chronologic age alone should not be a defining factor in treatment planning (Clayman et al., 1998; Kagan et al., 2002). The role of healthcare professionals is to empower older individuals to make appropriate choices in terms of living with cancer and then support them in their individual choices (Thome, Dykes, Gunnars, & Hallberg, 2003).

Stage

Patients with head and neck cancer most often present with complaints of a mass, otalgia, dysphagia, pain, or bleeding. Cervical adenopathy may be present as well. Once the diagnosis has been established, the tumor is staged, specific to the primary site, according to the tumor-node-metastasis classification system developed by the American Joint Committee on Cancer (Harris, 2000). Disease stage usually dictates the treatment modality and also is a useful prognostic indicator (Forastiere et al., 1998).

Treatment Modalities

Current treatment modalities for head and neck cancer include surgical resection, often with reconstruction, radiation therapy, and chemotherapy. A single modality (e.g., surgery, radiation) can be used for early-stage tumors. However, combined modalities usually are required for advanced tumors (Spaulding, 2002).

Summary

Caring for the patient with head and neck cancer presents tremendous nursing challenges in all practice settings. Today, improved surgical techniques combined with conservative treatment approaches are leading to more favorable outcomes with improved function, cosmesis, and symptom management. Oncology nurses play a critical role in coordinating patient care and providing appropriate interventions and patient education.

References

Allison, P., Franco, E., Black, M., & Feine, J. (1998). The role of professional diagnostic delays in the prognosis of upper aerodigestive tract carcinoma. *Oral Oncology, 34,* 147–153.

American Cancer Society. (1996). *Cancer statistics for African Americans, 1996.* Atlanta, GA: Author.

Aubertin, M.A. (1997). Oral cancer screening in the elderly: The home healthcare nurse's role. *Home Healthcare Nurse, 15,* 595–604.

Barroso, J., McMillan, S., Casey, L., Gibson, W., Kaminski, G., & Meyer, J. (2000). Comparison between African-American and white women in their beliefs about breast cancer and their health locus of control. *Cancer Nursing, 23,* 268–276.

Blot, W.J. (1992). Alcohol and cancer. *Cancer Research, 52*(Suppl. 7), 2119S–2123S.

Clayman, G.L., Eicher, S.A., Sicard, M.W., Razmpa, E., & Goepfert, H. (1998). Surgical outcomes in head and neck cancer patients 80 years of age and older. *Head and Neck, 20,* 216–223.

Dessner, S.H. (2000). Prevention and detection. In A.S. Luggen & S.E. Meiner (Eds.), *Handbook for the care of the older adult with cancer* (pp. 9–24). Pittsburgh, PA: Oncology Nursing Society.

Dropkin, M.J. (1999). Head and neck cancer: A recovery perspective. *Developments in Supportive Cancer Care, 3,* 49–52.

Forastiere, A., Goepfert, H., Goffinet, D., Hong, K.W., Laramore, G., Mittal, B., et al. (1998). NCCN practice guidelines for head and neck cancer. National Comprehensive Cancer Network. *Oncology, 12*(7A), 39–147.

Foxall, M., Barron, C., & Houfek, J. (2001). Ethnic influences on body awareness, trait anxiety, perceived risk, and breast and gynecologic cancer screening practices. *Oncology Nursing Forum, 28,* 727–738.

Friedlander, P., Schantz, S., Shaha, A., Yu, G., & Shah, J. (1998). Squamous cell carcinoma of the tongue in young patients: A matched-pair analysis. *Head and Neck, 20,* 363–368.

Guidry, J., Greisinger, A., Aday, L.A., Winn, R.J., Vernon, S., & Throckmorton, T.A. (1996). Barriers to cancer treatment: A review of published research. *Oncology Nursing Forum, 23,* 1393–1398.

Harris, L.L. (2000). Head and neck malignancies. In C.H. Yarbro, M.H. Frogge, M. Goodman, & S.L. Groenwald (Eds.), *Cancer nursing: Principles and practice* (5th ed., pp. 1210–1243). Sudbury, MA: Jones and Bartlett.

Hirano, M., & Mori, K. (1998). Management of cancer in the elderly: Therapeutic dilemmas. *Otolaryngology—Head and Neck Surgery, 118,* 110–114.

Jemal, A., Murray, T., Ward, E., Samuels, A., Tiwari, R., Ghafoor, A., et al. (2005). Cancer statistics, 2005. *CA: A Cancer Journal for Clinicians, 55,* 10–30.

Jones, A., Beasley, N., Houghton, D., & Husband, D. (1998). The effects of age on survival and other parameters in squamous cell carcinoma of the oral cavity, pharynx and larynx. *Clinical Otolaryngology, 23,* 51–56.

Kagan, S.H., Chalian, A.A., Goldberg, A.N., Rontal, M.L., Weinstein, G.S., Prior, B., et al. (2002). Impact of age on clinical care pathway length of stay following complex head and neck resection. *Head and Neck, 24,* 545–548.

Khuri, F., Kim, E.S., Lee, J.J., Winn, R.J., Benner, S.E., Lippman, S.M., et al. (2001). The impact of smoking status, disease stage, and index tumor site on second primary tumor incidence and tumor recurrence in the head and neck retinoid chemoprevention trial. *Cancer Epidemiology, Biomarkers and Prevention, 10,* 823–829.

Montgomery, W.W., Lazor, J.B., & Weber, A.L. (2002). Anatomy, examination, and diagnosis. In W.W. Montgomery (Ed.), *Surgery of the larynx, trachea, esophagus and neck* (pp. 1–42). Philadelphia: W.B. Saunders.

Mood, D.W. (1997). Cancers of the head and neck. In C. Varricchio (Ed.), *A cancer source book for nurses* (7th ed., pp. 271–283). Atlanta, GA: American Cancer Society.

Paterson, I.C., Eveson, J., & Prime, S.S. (1996). Molecular changes in oral cancer may reflect aetiology and ethnic origin. *European Journal of Cancer, Oral Oncology, 32B,* 150–153.

Patten, C.A., Martin, J.E., & Owen, N. (1996). Can psychiatric and chemical dependency treatment units be smoke free? *Journal of Substance Abuse Treatment, 13,* 107–118.

Phillips, J., Cohen, M., & Moses, G. (1999). Breast cancer screening and African American women: Fear, fatalism, and silence. *Oncology Nursing Forum, 26,* 561–571.

Robinson, K., Kimmel, E., & Yasko, J. (1995). Reaching out to the African American community through innovative strategies. *Oncology Nursing Forum, 22,* 1383–1391.

Rose, P., & Yates, P. (2001). Quality of life experienced by patients receiving radiation treatment for cancers of the head and neck. *Cancer Nursing, 24,* 255–263.

Scully, C., & Porter, S. (2000). Oral cancer. *BMJ, 321,* 97–100.

Singh, B., Bhaya, M., Zimbler, M., Stern, J., Roland, J., Rosenfeld, R., et al. (1998). Impact of co-morbidity on young patients with head and neck squamous cell carcinoma. *Head and Neck, 20,* 1–7.

Spaulding, M.B. (2002). Recent advances in the treatment of head and neck cancer: A patient care perspective. *ORL—Head and Neck Nursing, 20*(1), 9–15.

Thome, B., Dykes, A., Gunnars, B., & Hallberg, I.R. (2003). The experiences of older people living with cancer. *Cancer Nursing, 26,* 85–96.

U.S. Department of Health and Human Services. (2000, July). *Tobacco use among U.S. racial/ethnic minority groups—African Americans, American Indians and Alaska Natives, Asian Americans and Pacific Islanders, and Hispanics: A report of the surgeon general.* Retrieved November 19, 2004, from http://www.cdc.gov/tobacco/sgr/sgr_1998/

CHAPTER 2

Anatomy and Physiology

Joan Such Lockhart, PhD, RN, CORLN, AOCN®, FAAN, and
Lenore K. Resick, MSN, CRNP, BC, NP-C, Doctoral Candidate

Introduction

This chapter provides an overview of ear, nose, throat, and head and neck anatomy and physiology. Head and neck cancer and its medical and surgical treatments often alter the structure of these anatomic features and impact their associated functions: hearing, balance, smell, taste, breathing, mastication, swallowing, and speaking. Assessing these changes is essential in developing an appropriate plan of care and optimal patient outcomes.

The Ear

The ear consists of three anatomic regions: the external ear, the middle ear, and the inner ear (see Figure 2-1). The external ear is the visible portion and extends inward to the lateral surface of the tympanic membrane. The external ear consists of two major structures, the auricle (pinna) and the external auditory (ear) canal, which also is known as the acoustic meatus. The auricle houses several landmark structures: the helix, tragus, antitragus, and lobule. The external auditory canal is located near the temporomandibular joint anteriorly and the parotid gland inferiorly (see Figure 2-2).

The auricle and external auditory canal direct sound waves toward the tympanic membrane. The length and shape of the canal and the direction of hair follicles lining the canal protect the tympanic membrane and middle ear from trauma and foreign bodies (Seeley, Stephens, & Tate, 1998). In children, the external ear canal curves upward and is shorter than the external ear canal of an adult (Alvord & Farmer, 1997).

Figure 2-1. External, Middle, and Inner Ear

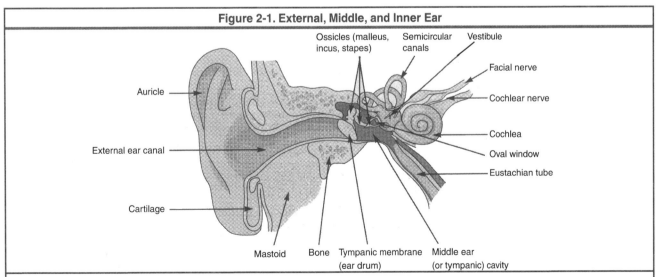

Note. From "Normal Anatomy and Physiology" (p. 43), by H.G. Andresen, M.H. Cyr, J.P. Guadagnini, M.M. Hickey, T.S. Higgins, M.B. Huntoon, et al. in L.L. Harris and M.B. Huntoon (Eds.), *Core Curriculum for Otorhinolaryngology and Head-Neck Nursing,* 1998, New Smyrna Beach, FL: Society of Otorhinolaryngology and Head-Neck Nurses, Inc. Copyright 1998 by Society of Otorhinolaryngology and Head-Neck Nurses, Inc. Reprinted with permission.

Figure 2-2. Cross-Section of the External, Middle, and Inner Ear in Relationship to Other Structures of the Head and Face

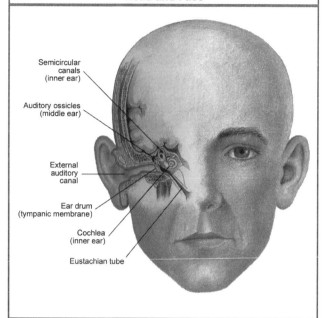

Semicircular canals (inner ear)

Auditory ossicles (middle ear)

External auditory canal

Ear drum (tympanic membrane)

Cochlea (inner ear)

Eustachian tube

Note. From *Mosby's Guide to Physical Examination* (4th ed., p. 309), by H.M. Seidel, J.W. Ball, J.E. Dains, and G.W. Benedict, 1999, St. Louis, MO: Mosby. Copyright 1999 by Mosby. Reprinted with permission.

The cartilaginous outer lateral region of the ear canal is covered with thick skin, and the bony two-thirds inner medial region is lined with thin skin and is very sensitive to pain. The outer lateral aspect of the ear canal contains hair follicles and glands that contribute to the formation of cerumen.

Lymph drainage from the external auditory canal flows anteriorly to the preauricular lymph nodes, interiorly to the deep upper cervical nodes, and posteriorly to the lymph nodes in the mastoid region.

The middle ear is an air-filled space located in the temporal bone of the head. The tympanic membrane, a translucent, pearly gray membrane, marks the end of the external auditory canal and the beginning of the middle ear. When sound waves from the environment hit against the tympanic membrane, the membrane vibrates, transmitting these vibrations to the three small bones of the middle ear: the malleus, incus, and stapes (Duckert, 1998). These vibrations cause the stapes to move at the oval window of the inner ear. This results in vibration of the oval window, which causes movement of fluids in the inner ear.

For the tympanic membrane to vibrate, the atmospheric pressure both inside and outside the ear must be equal. The eustachian tube, which extends from the middle ear to the nasopharynx, equalizes the atmospheric pressure. The eustachian tube permits air to flow to or from the middle ear,

allowing the air pressure of the environment to equal that of the middle ear.

The inner ear contains the facial nerve (cranial nerve VII) and the neuroreceptor organs responsible for balance and hearing. Both balance and hearing are transmitted to the brain by the acoustic (vestibulocochlear) nerve (cranial nerve VIII), which has a vestibular and cochlear division. "Vestibular" refers to the inner ear and the vestibule that is responsible for balance. "Cochlear" refers to the cochlea of the inner ear and is responsible for hearing. The structures of the inner ear lie within the protective cavity of the temporal bone.

The Nose and Paranasal Sinuses

The nose consists of an outer portion and an inner portion (see Figure 2-3). The framework of the nose consists of nasal bones and portions of the superior maxillary bone. Cartilage comprises the upper and lateral portions of the nose and the nasal septum. This bony and cartilaginous structure makes up the nasal cavities. The nasal cavities open anteriorly by two pear-shaped nares (nostrils) and posteriorly through openings into the nasopharynx. Soft tissue and skin cover the outside of the nose. The region that is slightly dilated and lies just inside the nose is the nasal vestibule. The vestibule extends into the tip of the nose.

Olfactory and respiratory regions comprise the areas above and behind the nasal vestibule. The frontal sinus, sphenoid sinus, and cribriform plate make up the supralateral boundary of the nose. Inside the nose, the nasal cavity is divided by the nasal septum into two chambers and consists of the vestibule, septum, roof, floor, cribriform, and turbinates or lateral walls (see Figure 2-4).

The nose receives an extensive blood supply from several branches of the internal and external carotid arteries: the posterior ethmoid arteries, posterior septal nasal arteries, major palatine artery, anterior ethmoid artery, and the septal

Figure 2-3. Anatomic Structures of the External Nose

Bridge

Tip

Columella

Anterior naris (nostril)

Vestibule

Ala nasi

Figure 2-4. Cross-Sectional View of the Anatomic Structures of the Nose and Nasopharynx

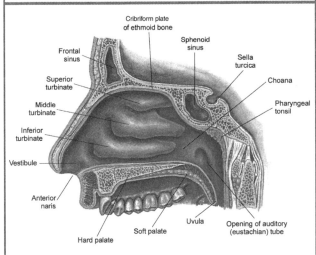

Cribriform plate of ethmoid bone
Sphenoid sinus
Frontal sinus
Sella turcica
Superior turbinate
Choana
Middle turbinate
Pharyngeal tonsil
Inferior turbinate
Vestibule
Anterior naris
Uvula
Opening of auditory (eustachian) tube
Hard palate
Soft palate

Note. From *Mosby's Guide to Physical Examination* (4th ed., p. 312), by H.M. Seidel, J.W. Ball, J.E. Dains, and G.W. Benedict, 1999, St. Louis, MO: Mosby. Copyright 1999 by Mosby. Reprinted with permission.

branch of the superior labial artery. Several smaller arteries join together to form a network of vessels on the nasal septum in the anterior portion of the nose called Kiesselbach plexus or Little area (Andresen et al., 1998).

The nose protects the lungs by filtering, warming, and moisturizing the air that is inhaled. As air passes through the nasal cavities, it is warmed and moistened by the surfaces of the nasal turbinates and nasal septum. The inhaled air is filtered by coarse hairs (vibrissae) in the nasal mucosa and by precipitation of particles on the turbinates (Schwab & Zenkel, 1998).

The nose contains the olfactory nerve (cranial nerve I) endings and serves as the peripheral organ involved in the sense of smell, which also augments the sense of taste. The olfactory receptors lie within the olfactory membrane located high in the nose and originate from the central nervous system.

The paranasal sinuses are named after the skull bones in which they are located: the frontal, ethmoid, maxillary, and sphenoid sinuses (see Figure 2-5). Each sinus is paired. These four sets of air-filled sinuses are lined with ciliated respiratory mucosa, which contains mucus-producing cells. The mucosal lining of all the paranasal sinuses is continuous with that of the mucosa of the nasal cavity.

The paranasal sinuses serve several functions. The paranasal sinuses protect the brain against frontal trauma by absorbing shock and providing insulation. They help to humidify and warm inhaled air by adding to the surface area of the olfactory membrane. The sinuses also play a role with voice resonance and are thought to aid in the growth of the

face without adding to the weight of the skull bones (Graney & Baker, 1998).

The Oral Cavity and Salivary Glands

The mouth consists of two parts, the vestibule and the oral cavity (see Figure 2-6). The vestibule is the narrow space that is bordered on the outside by the lips and cheeks and on the inside by the gingivae and teeth. The oral cavity is surrounded at its anterior and lateral sides by the alveolar arches, teeth, and gingivae and on its posterior side by the oropharynx. The palate borders the oral cavity superiorly, and most of the tongue's base forms the oral cavity's inferior border or the floor of the mouth. The oral cavity is lined with simple, moist columnar epithelium that is continuous with the lining of the oropharynx. The floor of the mouth is extremely vascular.

The oral cavity contains several structures that play a key role in respiration, mastication, swallowing, and speech production. Structures in the mouth that are key to these functions include the lips, cheeks, buccal mucosa, teeth, gums, tongue, hard palate, and soft palate. The mouth also houses the openings of ducts that connect with the salivary glands.

Figure 2-5. Paranasal Sinuses: Anterior View of Skull and Left Lateral View of Skull

Frontal sinus
Sphenoidal sinus
Frontal sinus
Ethmoid sinus cell
Maxillary sinus
Nasal septum

Note. Copyright 2000 by WebMD. Reprinted with permission.

Figure 2-6. Anatomic Structures of the Oral Cavity

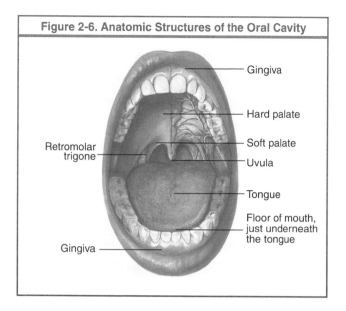

Lips, Cheeks, and Buccal Mucosa

Both the lips and cheeks are constructed of skeletal muscle covered with skin. The orbicularis oris muscle that inserts in the corners of the mouth forms the bulk of the superior and inferior lips. The buccinator muscles form the bulk of the cheeks and insert into the maxilla and mandible. Externally, the lips appear as dark or reddened areas that are distinctly different in color from the facial skin that surrounds them. This coloring results from capillary blood that shows through the translucent epithelium covering of the lips. A visible margin called the vermilion cutaneous line separates this dark region of the lips from the face. Receptors help the lips to sense both the texture and temperature of food or objects with which they come into contact.

Inside the oral cavity, the lips are lined with poorly keratinized mucous membrane that is continuous with the lining of the mouth. A small extension of mucous membrane lining, the labial frenulum, joins the inside of each lip with the mouth lining. The inside portion of the cheeks is referred to as the buccal mucosa. In addition to the buccinator muscles, these lateral walls contain adipose tissue, areolar tissue, blood vessels, and glands that secrete mucus. The space that forms a trough between the lips, cheeks, and teeth is the vestibule.

The lips close to keep food and fluid in the oral cavity during mastication. The cheeks and buccal mucosa help to control the location of food while it is between the teeth and in the oral cavity and secure the food as the teeth break and grind it into smaller pieces. During speech, the lips help with articulation. Both the lips and cheeks contribute to the animation of the face as it changes expressions for such actions as kissing, smiling, and frowning through the action of the facial nerve (cranial nerve VII). The trigeminal nerve (cranial nerve V) allows for the jaw to clench as it provides the motor supply to the temporal and masseter muscles. The trigeminal nerve also permits the jaw to move laterally (Andresen et al., 1998).

Teeth and Gingiva

The teeth are positioned in alveoli, or sockets, located within the processes of the maxilla and mandible. These alveolar ridges are covered by gingivae, dense fibrous connective tissue layered with stratified squamous epithelium. The teeth are held firmly in place by periodontal ligaments and cementum, a bone-like substance produced by the periodontal membrane that lines the alveoli. The teeth are innervated by branches of the trigeminal nerve (cranial nerve V), specifically, the superior and inferior alveolar nerves. Branches of the maxillary artery, the superior and inferior alveolar arteries, supply blood to the teeth.

The cutting, tearing, grinding, and crushing abilities of the teeth make them instrumental during mastication. This mechanical action of the teeth turns large bites of food into small pieces that can be mixed readily with saliva, broken down by digestive enzymes, and easily swallowed. The teeth also play an important role in the articulation of various sounds during speech.

Tongue

The tongue extends from its anterior tip, or apex, which is visible through the opening of the oral cavity, to its posterior attachment, or base in the oropharynx. The tongue occupies most of the oral cavity. The anterior two-thirds of the tongue is attached by its undersurface to the floor of the mouth by a fold of mucous membrane called the lingual frenulum. The posterior one-third of the tongue continues toward the oropharynx, where it is attached by mucous membranes (see Figure 2-7).

The tongue itself is a large muscular structure constructed of interlocking skeletal fibers. The dorsal surface of the tongue is covered with three types of papillae that are small extensions of the tongue's mucosa: fungiform, filiform, and circumvallate. Fungiform papillae contain the receptors for taste, called taste buds. Filiform papillae lack taste buds but provide the tongue with a rough surface that assists with eating and chewing. A third type of papillae, circumvallate papillae, is positioned directly in front of the sulcus terminalis near the back portion of the tongue and contains taste buds. The remaining dorsal surface of the posterior tongue lacks papillae but contains a few taste buds as well as a mass of lymph tissue called the lingual tonsil. The ventral side, or undersurface, of the tongue has a relatively smooth appearance. The ducts of the submandibular glands drain saliva in this area, near the lingual frenulum.

The tongue plays a vital role in mastication and in the initial phases of swallowing. As food enters the mouth, the tongue positions the food and allows the food to be chewed and broken down into smaller particles by the teeth. The tongue moves its position within the mouth and changes its shape to allow food particles to mix with saliva. The taste buds provide the many sensations associated with eating. The facial nerve (cranial nerve VII) provides taste sensation to the anterior two-thirds of the tongue (salty, sweet, sour, and bitter), whereas the glossopharyngeal nerve (cranial nerve IX) provides these taste sensations to the posterior tongue (Bickley & Szilagyi, 2003).

The tongue actively moves the chewed bolus of food toward the oropharynx to be swallowed. To do this, the tongue elevates within the mouth and contracts against the hard palate, pushing the food toward the back of the pharynx. The tongue also plays a significant role in communication. The mobility of the tongue provides articulation and facilitates pronunciation of words, specifically consonants such as D, K, and T.

Hard and Soft Palates

The palate forms the roof of the mouth (see Figure 2-6). The entire palate consists of two continuous portions, the anterior hard palate and the posterior soft palate. The uvula, a small piece of tissue hanging inferiorly from the midline edge of the soft palate, easily can locate the soft palate.

A thick layer of rough mucosa covers the hard palate, which is marked by a midline ridge (palatine raphe). The soft palate connects to the tongue and oropharyngeal wall by two

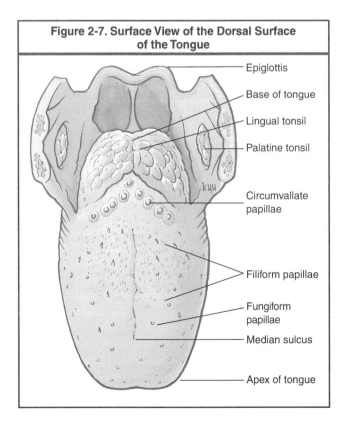

Figure 2-7. Surface View of the Dorsal Surface of the Tongue

- Epiglottis
- Base of tongue
- Lingual tonsil
- Palatine tonsil
- Circumvallate papillae
- Filiform papillae
- Fungiform papillae
- Median sulcus
- Apex of tongue

vertical pairs of folds, the anterior and posterior pillars. These folds, the soft palate, and the uvula form an arch above and posterior to the tongue. The opening of this arch is referred to as the fauces. The palatine tonsils lie in the fossae between the anterior and posterior pillars.

Like the tongue, the hard and soft palates play an important role in mastication, swallowing, and speech production. The hard palate provides a firm, rough surface against which the tongue can move food particles as they gradually mix with saliva. The soft palate moves upward and closes the entrance to the nasopharynx. This action prevents food and fluids from entering the nasopharynx during swallowing. The movement of the soft palate is considered an involuntary reflex action rather than a voluntary conscious movement, as with the tongue. As food moves into the oropharynx, the soft palate returns to its resting position, allowing normal respiration to resume.

Salivary Glands

Three major pairs of salivary glands exist: parotid, submandibular (submaxillary), and sublingual (see Figure 2-8). The main purpose of these glands is to produce saliva, with the submandibular gland secreting the majority (more than two-thirds). Each set of glands has its specific lymphatic network that drains into lymph nodes in the head and neck region.

The parotid glands are the largest pair of salivary glands, located superficially behind the mandible and directly below and anterior to the ears. Branches of the facial nerve (cranial nerve VII) divide the parotid gland into a superficial lobe and a deep lobe, connected by tissue referred to as the isthmus. The superficial lobe is larger than the deep lobe. Stenson's ducts drain saliva from the parotid glands and open into the oral mucosa in the vestibule, next to the second upper molars.

The submandibular (submaxillary) glands are the second-largest salivary glands, located near the inner surface of the mandible. Wharton's ducts carry saliva to the mouth and open on the floor of the mouth on either side of the frenulum.

The sublingual glands are the smallest pair of salivary glands. They are located under the mucosa of the floor of the mouth under the tongue and anterior to the submandibular gland. The sublingual glands contain approximately 5–15 ducts that drain saliva into the floor of the mouth (Shidnia & Hornback, 1999).

Saliva is more than 99% water, slightly acidic (pH 6.8), and hypotonic (Shidnia & Hornback, 1999). Saliva contains several substances, including electrolytes, amylase, proteins such as mucin, lysozyme, IgA, and waste products from the body's metabolism (Marieb, 1998). These substances not only aid with digestion and prevent tooth decay but also protect the body against invading microorganisms.

Saliva helps individuals to accomplish several key processes, such as digestion, taste, swallowing, and speech. In addition to these functions, saliva also protects the oral

Figure 2-8. The Salivary Glands, Shown in Left Lateral View

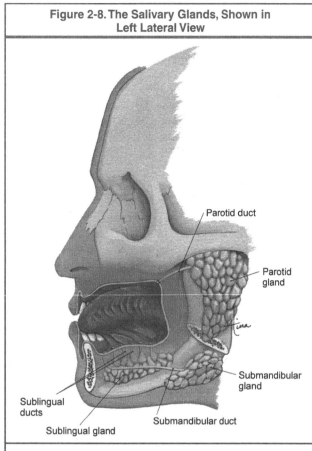

Parotid duct

Parotid gland

Submandibular gland

Submandibular duct

Sublingual ducts

Sublingual gland

Note. From *Essentials of Anatomy and Physiology* (3rd ed., p. 355), by V.C. Scanlon and T. Sanders, 1999, Philadelphia: F.A. Davis. Copyright 1999 by F.A. Davis. Reprinted with permission.

structures against invasion by microorganisms. Saliva assists with digestion through its enzyme amylase that breaks down ingested carbohydrates into smaller chains of glucose molecules or maltose. As a person chews food, chemicals in the food become dissolved in the saliva. This process enables the taste buds in the fungiform papillae of the tongue to sense various tastes. Saliva moistens the food particles and allows them to adhere together into a ball or bolus. This bolus then moves toward the pharynx to be swallowed. Because saliva acts as a lubricant in the mouth, it also facilitates the production of speech. Moistened with saliva, the tongue, lips, and teeth can move freely within the oral cavity so that words can be pronounced (Andresen et al., 1998).

Pharynx

The pharynx is a funnel-shaped passageway that connects the nasal cavity with the larynx and the mouth with the esophagus (see Figure 2-9). The superior end of the pharynx begins at the base of the skull and extends downward for approximately

12 cm (4.7 inches) to the level of the larynx near the sixth cervical vertebra (McMinn, Hutchings, & Logan, 1994).

The pharynx consists anatomically of three primary regions: the nasopharynx, oropharynx, and laryngopharynx (hypopharynx). Each of these regions of the pharynx contains vital structures that play an important role in breathing, swallowing, and speaking.

The pharynx serves several purposes related to breathing and swallowing. Except for its most superior region, the nasopharynx, which transports air, the pharynx is a common pathway for air, food, and fluids. As a person inspires air through the nose and/or mouth, it travels downward through the pharynx. As air travels to the lungs, it passes through the larynx, trachea, and right and left bronchi. When a person ingests food or fluids through the mouth, the pharynx channels the food bolus downward through the esophagus toward the stomach. Unlike in the mouth, no digestion takes place in the pharynx. The muscles of the pharynx assist with sound production and speech by changing the shape of the pharynx.

Nasopharynx

The most superior portion of the pharynx, the nasopharynx, is located behind the nose and nasal cavity and in front of the sphenoid bone. The nasopharynx starts at the base of the skull inferior to the sphenoid bone and extends down-

Figure 2-9. Midsagittal Section of the Head and Neck, Showing the Structures of the Upper Respiratory Tract

Nasal septum

Nasal cavity

Palate

Tongue

Nasopharynx

Oropharynx

Laryngopharynx (hypopharynx)

ward to the lower border of the soft palate. The lining of the nasopharynx is continuous with that of the nose and nasal cavity. The pseudostratified columnar epithelium lining of the nasopharynx contains cilia that assist with removal of mucus and secretions.

Because the nasopharynx is located above the mouth, it serves as a passageway for the transport of air but not food. During the swallowing process, the inferior opening of the nasopharynx is sealed off by the upward movement of the soft palate and uvula. This protective mechanism prevents food from entering the nasopharynx during swallowing.

The nasopharynx houses two important structures, the pharyngeal tonsils and the openings of the auditory (pharyngotympanic or eustachian) tubes. Each of these structures is paired. The pharyngeal tonsils, commonly referred to as adenoids when enlarged, are clumps of lymphoid tissue positioned high on the posterior wall of the nasopharynx behind the nasal cavity.

Oropharynx

The oropharynx, the middle segment of the pharynx, starts at the inferior end of the nasopharynx. The oropharynx lies behind the oral cavity and is continuous with it. The oropharynx extends superiorly from the soft palate and extends downward to the upper border of the epiglottis. Unlike the nasopharynx, the oropharynx serves as a passage for both air and food.

The lining of the oropharynx differs from that of the nasopharynx. Its stratified squamous epithelium lining helps to protect the oropharynx from mechanical and chemical irritation caused by food and fluids that come into contact with it during swallowing.

The oropharynx houses two additional tonsils, the palatine and the lingual tonsils. The pair of palatine tonsils is embedded in the lateral mucosal walls between the two sets of arches in the oral cavity and is larger in size than the adenoids. The lingual tonsil is not paired and covers the base of the tongue. Combined, these tonsils in the oropharynx together with the pharyngeal tonsils of the nasopharynx comprise a circle of lymphatic tissue called Waldeyer ring that serves as an initial line of defense against pathogens that enter the pharynx (Andresen et al., 1998).

Laryngopharynx (Hypopharynx)

A third segment of the pharynx is the laryngopharynx, or hypopharynx, located behind the epiglottis and extending from the level of the hyoid bone to the lower edge of the cricoid cartilage of the larynx, level with the sixth cervical vertebra. The laryngopharynx is located behind the larynx and partially encircles it on either side. Like the oropharynx, the laryngopharynx is a common passageway for both food and air. These two pathways separate at the level of the larynx. Food and fluids travel from the laryngopharynx through the esophagus to the stomach. Air passes through the structures

of the larynx downward through the trachea, bronchi, and lungs. This movement of air is delayed to permit swallowing to occur.

The laryngopharynx consists of pharyngeal walls, the pyriform sinuses, and the postcricoid area. The pyriform sinus is a space located on each side of the thyroid cartilage in the larynx. The laryngopharynx is continuous with the oropharynx superiorly and esophagus inferiorly. The lining of the laryngopharynx is similar to that of the oropharynx, stratified squamous epithelium. The laryngopharynx has a rich supply of lymphatics.

The larynx connects the pharynx with the trachea. The larynx lies between the fourth and sixth cervical vertebrae and is approximately 5 cm (2 inches) long (Marieb, 1998). The larynx is attached from the hyoid bone at the level of the third cervical vertebra superiorly, opens into the laryngopharynx, and is continuous with the trachea inferiorly.

The larynx serves important functions related to breathing, swallowing, and speech production. First, cartilages of the larynx keep the airway open so that air exchange can occur during respiration. Second, the larynx prevents aspiration of food, fluids, and saliva during swallowing through the protective actions of the epiglottis and vocal cords. The larynx enables the cough reflex and Valsalva maneuver (bearing down against a closed glottis) to occur. Third, the larynx aids with phonation by creating sounds through vibrations of the vocal cords.

The hyoid bone lies just above the larynx at the level of the third cervical vertebra but is not considered part of the larynx. It is attached to the larynx by muscles and membranes and supports the base of the tongue (see Figure 2-10).

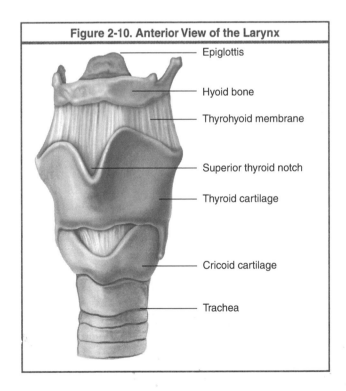

Figure 2-10. Anterior View of the Larynx

Epiglottis

Hyoid bone

Thyrohyoid membrane

Superior thyroid notch

Thyroid cartilage

Cricoid cartilage

Trachea

The larynx is composed of a framework of nine cartilages, three that are single (unpaired) and three that are paired. The single cartilages of the larynx are the thyroid cartilage, the cricoid cartilage, and the epiglottis. The thyroid cartilage lies at the level of the fourth and fifth cervical vertebra and is shaped like a shield. The thyroid cartilage is commonly referred to as the "Adam's apple" because of its midline laryngeal prominence that often is evident on a person's neck. The angle of this prominence is more obvious in males than in females because of sex hormones secreted in males during adolescence.

The cricoid cartilage lies directly beneath the thyroid cartilage at the level of the sixth cervical vertebra and is shaped like a signet ring, with the band (arch) at the front and the stone (lamina) at the back of the larynx. The cricoid is the only cartilage that entirely encircles the larynx. This thick cartilage is one of the most important of all laryngeal cartilages and provides the base for many laryngeal functions. The cricoid cartilage marks the beginning of the trachea.

The leaf-shaped epiglottis is attached to the anterior edge of the thyroid cartilage and extends superiorly to the back portion of the tongue. During swallowing, the larynx moves upward and the epiglottis tips over the larynx to shield the opening. This action of the epiglottis prevents food, fluids, and saliva from entering the larynx. If food or fluids enter the larynx, the protective cough reflex voluntarily initiates to help the body to expel the substance. During quiet respiration, the superior flap of the epiglottis extends upward, allowing air to pass freely through the larynx.

Three smaller sets of paired cartilages—the arytenoid, cuneiform, and corniculate cartilages—comprise a portion of the lateral and posterior laryngeal walls. Two pairs of ligaments stretch from the anterior side of the arytenoid cartilage to the posterior surface of the thyroid cartilage. The most superior pair of ligaments is called the false vocal cords or the vestibular folds. The false vocal cords do not play a direct role in sound production but help to protect the airway.

The inferior pair of ligaments, two V-shaped bands of elastic tissue, form the true vocal cords, or vocal folds. These vocal cords lie directly beneath the thyroid cartilage and above the cricoid cartilage. The space between the vocal cords is referred to as the glottis. During quiet breathing, the vocal cords remain apart to permit the flow of air to and from the lungs through the glottis. The vocal cords are the primary structures responsible for producing speech and sound.

The true vocal cords come together to allow a person to perform a Valsalva maneuver, in which expired air is forced against a closed glottis, mouth, or nose. This maneuver is useful in a variety of everyday activities, such as lifting heavy objects or having a bowel movement. The vagus nerve (cranial nerve X) provides the motor supply to the palate, pharynx, and larynx and sensation to the pharynx and larynx.

The larynx anatomically consists of three regions (superior to inferior) that are referred to in the classification and clinical treatment plan of laryngeal tumors: the supraglottis, glottis, and subglottis. The most superior segment of the larynx, the supraglottic region, extends from the epiglottis superiorly downward to the level of the true vocal cords. This area has a rich blood and lymphatic supply. The second segment of the larynx is the glottic region, which consists mainly of the true vocal cords. This region has a sparse blood and lymphatic supply. The third segment of the larynx, the subglottic region, starts just below the true vocal cords and extends inferiorly to the lower border of the cricoid cartilage. This region contains a rich lymphatic supply.

The lining of the larynx is continuous with that of the pharynx. The larynx is lined with pseudostratified ciliated columnar epithelium that helps to remove both mucus and debris. Stratified squamous epithelium covers both the false and true vocal cords.

The larynx receives its blood supply from the laryngeal and cricothyroid arteries, branches of the external carotid, and common carotid arteries. The laryngeal and thyroid veins drain blood from the head and neck and return it to the heart via the internal jugular vein. The larynx receives most of its motor and sensory supply from the recurrent laryngeal nerve and the superior laryngeal nerves.

Trachea

The trachea is a 10–12-cm (4–4.8-inch) tube approximately 2.5 cm (1 inch) in diameter (Marieb, 1998; Sigler & Schuring, 1993) that lies anterior to the esophagus and connects the larynx at the cricoid cartilage with both main stem bronchi and lungs. The walls of the trachea are supported with C-shaped hyaline cartilages.

Esophagus

The esophagus is a 25-cm (10-inch) tube that lies behind the trachea and connects the pharynx with the stomach (Marieb, 1998). The muscular walls of the esophagus remain collapsed unless its peristalsis moves food toward the stomach. Unlike in the oral cavity, no digestion of food occurs in the esophagus.

General Head and Neck Anatomy and Physiology

Skull and Facial Bones

The human skull consists of 22 bones, 8 cranial bones and 14 facial bones (Marieb, 1998). The uppermost portion of the skull is called the roof or skull cap (cranial vault); the floor of the cranial vault is referred to as the skull base. Three cavities exist within the skull: the cranial cavity, nasal cavity, and orbital cavities. The cranial cavity is formed by cranial bones and houses and protects the brain, eyeballs, and ears. The nasal septum divides the nasal cavity lengthwise into two halves. The two orbital cavities contain the eyeballs.

Eight bones, two paired and four unpaired, form the cranial cavity itself: frontal (1), parietal (2), temporal (2), occipital (1), sphenoid (1), and ethmoid (1). The frontal, parietal, temporal, and occipital bones form the top and sides of the cranium, and the sphenoid and ethmoid bones comprise the orbits and the floor of the skull base. The junctions between the bones of the cranium are immovable joints, commonly referred to as sutures.

The facial skeleton comprises the anterior portion of the skull. Fourteen facial bones exist, six paired and two unpaired: the mandible (1), condyloid joint (2), maxilla (2), zygomatic (2), nasal (2), lacrimal (2), palatine (2), and vomer (1).

The mandible is a horseshoe-shaped bone that houses the sockets for roots of the lower teeth. The mandible is movable and connects with the temporal bone at the condyloid joints. The maxillae contain the sockets for the roots of the upper teeth and form the anterior part of the hard palate. The zygomatic bones form the cheekbones and connect with the maxillae, temporal, and frontal bones. The nasal bones create the bridge of the nose. The lacrimal bones contain the opening in which the nasolacrimal duct transports tears from the lacrimal duct to the nasal cavity. The palatine bones form the posterior portion of the hard palate. The vomer bone lies behind the palatine bone and forms the inferior portion of the nasal cavity. The maxillae, frontal, sphenoid, and ethmoid bones house the air-filled paranasal sinuses and connect with the nose.

Major Neck Regions

For descriptive purposes, the neck consists of two sections, an anterior triangle and posterior triangle. Figure 2-11 illustrates these anatomic landmarks of the neck. The sternocleidomastoid muscle (SCM) divides both triangles and borders them as it extends obliquely from the mastoid area downward to the clavicle and the manubrium of the sternum.

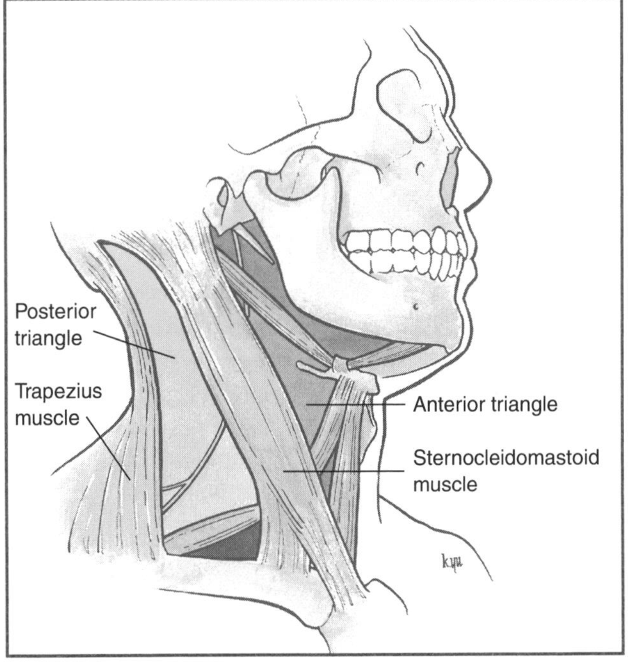

Major Blood Supply

Two pairs of major veins, the external and internal jugular veins, drain blood in the head and neck (see Figure 2-12). The external jugular vein runs diagonally over the surface of the SCM and drains blood from the superficial region of the posterior portions of the head and neck into the subclavian veins. The internal jugular veins lie deeper than the external veins and drain blood from the anterior portion of the face, head, neck, and venous sinuses of the cranial vault. The internal jugular veins connect with the subclavian veins to create the brachiocephalic veins.

Figure 2-11. Anterior and Posterior Triangles of the Neck

Posterior triangle
Trapezius muscle
Anterior triangle
Sternocleidomastoid muscle

Three vessels also drain into the brachiocephalic veins: the lingual veins, the superior thyroid veins, and the facial veins. The lingual veins drain the mouth and tongue, whereas the superior thyroid veins drain the thyroid and deep posterior face. The facial veins drain blood from the superior and anterior facial structures.

Blood that reaches the head and neck originates from three vessels that branch from the aortic arch: the brachiocephalic artery, the left common carotid artery, and the left subclavian artery. Each of these three arteries further separates into one or more smaller arteries as it approaches the structures of the face, head, and neck.

The first vessel, the brachiocephalic artery, separates at the level of the right clavicle into two vessels, the right subclavian artery and the right common carotid artery. The right subclavian artery provides blood to the upper part of the right arm but branches into the right vertebral artery that carries blood to the right brain. The right common carotid artery further divides into two vessels, the right external carotid artery and the right internal carotid artery. Branches of the right external carotid artery nourish the right side of the face, head, and neck region. Branches of the right internal carotid artery carry blood toward vessels that supply the right brain.

The second vessel, the left common carotid artery, extends from the aortic arch into two vessels, the left internal carotid artery and the left external carotid artery. The left internal carotid artery joins vessels that nourish the left brain. The left external carotid artery supplies blood to vessels that feed the left side of the face, head, and neck.

Figure 2-12. Underlying Structures of the Neck—Anterior View

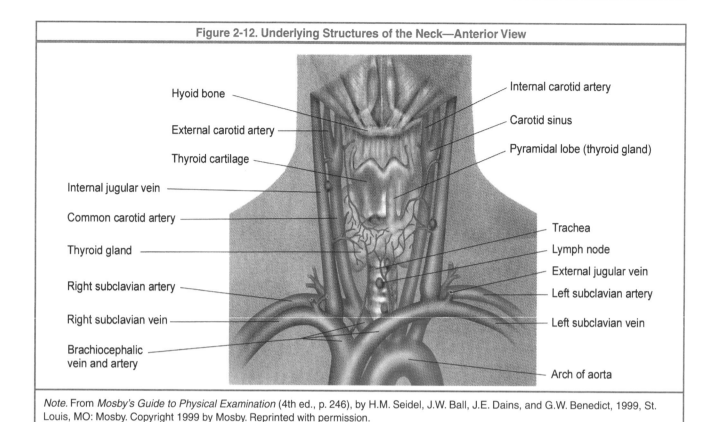

Hyoid bone

External carotid artery

Thyroid cartilage

Internal jugular vein

Common carotid artery

Thyroid gland

Right subclavian artery

Right subclavian vein

Brachiocephalic vein and artery

Internal carotid artery

Carotid sinus

Pyramidal lobe (thyroid gland)

Trachea

Lymph node

External jugular vein

Left subclavian artery

Left subclavian vein

Arch of aorta

Note. From *Mosby's Guide to Physical Examination* (4th ed., p. 246), by H.M. Seidel, J.W. Ball, J.E. Dains, and G.W. Benedict, 1999, St. Louis, MO: Mosby. Copyright 1999 by Mosby. Reprinted with permission.

The third vessel, the left subclavian artery, branches from the aortic arch to supply the upper portion of the left arm and divides into the left vertebral artery. Branches of the left vertebral artery supply blood to the left brain.

Major Muscle Groups

The head and neck region contains several major muscle groups that enable movement of the face, head, tongue, neck, and shoulders. The SCM of the anterior and lateral neck and the trapezius muscle of the scapular region are two muscles that can be affected by diseases and treatments to the head and neck region.

The SCM extends from the upper sternum (manubrium) medially and the clavicle to the mastoid process behind the ear (see Figure 2-13). Contraction of the SCM on one side enables the head to rotate to the opposite side and extends the head. For example, contraction of the right SCM enables the head to turn toward the left side. If both SCM muscles contract, then the neck flexes. The trapezius muscle extends from the scapula, the clavicle, and the thoracic vertebrae to the occipital protuberance. The trapezius muscle allows the shoulders to raise, lower, and adduct/abduct and extends the head and neck. It also elevates, depresses, retracts, rotates, and fixes the scapula. The accessory nerve (cranial nerve XI) provides the SCM and trapezius muscles with their motor supply.

Figure 2-13. Muscles of the Neck—Anterior Superficial and Posterior Superficial

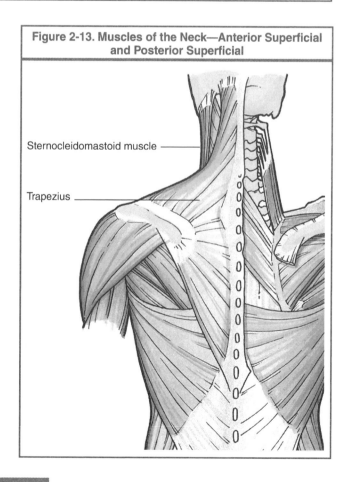

Sternocleidomastoid muscle

Trapezius

Lymphatic Supply and Cervical Lymph Nodes

The head and neck region contains a comprehensive lymphatic network that drains protein-rich fluid called lymph from the tissues of the body and returns it to the heart by way of the bloodstream. This connection between the lymphatic and circulatory systems is a closed one-way path, but a permeable one. Figure 2-14 illustrates the extensive lymphatic drainage system of the head and neck region.

Fluid drained from the interstitial spaces in the head and neck enters the microscopic and permeable lymph capillaries located near blood capillaries and travels through deep and superficial lymphatic collecting vessels. Lymph enters the cervical lymph nodes via afferent lymphatic vessels and exits using the efferent lymph vessels.

Cervical lymph nodes are superficial groups of nodes located along the lymphatic vessels on either side of the neck. The cervical nodes comprise one of the three sets of lymph nodes (along with inguinal and axillary nodes) in the body. Lymph nodes are small, measuring less than 1 cm. Some nodes are round, whereas others are oval or bean-shaped. A capsule made of thick fibrous tissue encases each node.

Lymph nodes defend the body through two mechanisms. First, cervical lymph nodes filter fluid drained from the head and neck region before returning it to the bloodstream, where it travels throughout the body. Macrophages in the nodes act as phagocytes, removing and destroying bacteria, viruses, and other harmful particles that enter the lymph fluid. Second, lymphocytes located in the nodes search the lymph fluid for antigens like bacteria, viruses, cancer cells, and other foreign bodies and destroy them before they have an opportunity to

harm the body. Because the flow of lymph fluid exiting the lymph node is slower than that entering the node, the lymph nodes have time to cleanse the lymph that passes through it. In addition to defending the body, the lymphatic system also helps the body to maintain its fluid balance and assists with the absorption of fats.

After being filtered by one or more lymph nodes, lymph passes through large collecting vessels called trunks into two lymphatic ducts on each side of the thoracic region, the right lymphatic duct and the left thoracic duct. The right lymphatic duct drains fluid from the right upper body. This includes the right side of the head and neck, the right portion of the upper arm, and the right side of the chest. The thoracic duct drains lymph from the left side of the head and neck and the remaining portions of the body.

Cervical lymph nodes undergo various changes as they encounter infections and cancer. For example, superficial lymph nodes become swollen and painful if they are obstructed as they destroy the many microscopic organisms that enter the lymph fluid. These nodes also swell without pain as cancer cells separate from a malignant tumor in the body, enter the lymphatic system, and become trapped in the nodes. In this situation, lymph nodes basically provide a route for cancer cells to spread to other sites in the body. Finally, diseases or surgery can cause the lymphatic ducts of regional lymph nodes to become obstructed or infected. This condition can result in a severe localized swelling of the area drained by the affected nodes called lymphedema. Enlarged cervical lymph nodes or neck masses, known as lymphadenopathy, frequently result from reactive hyperplasia, infection, metastatic tumors, or lymphoma.

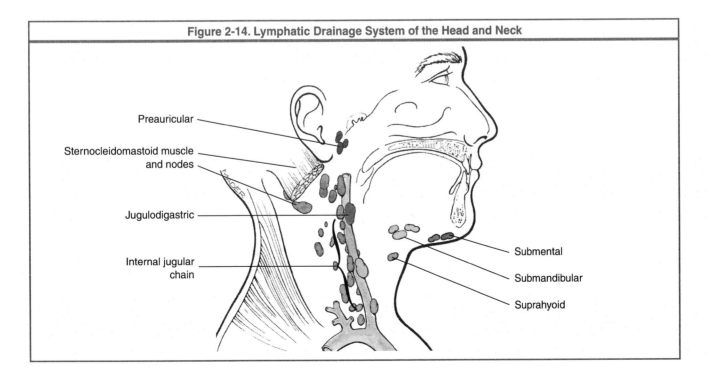

Figure 2-14. Lymphatic Drainage System of the Head and Neck

Preauricular

Sternocleidomastoid muscle and nodes

Jugulodigastric

Internal jugular chain

Submental

Submandibular

Suprahyoid

The appearance of lymph fluid varies in color, including clear, opaque, or yellow-tinged. Lymph fluid that is drained from the digestive viscera is referred to as chyle and appears milky white because it contains digested fats. Lymph also contains other substances extracted from the plasma and cells of the body, including water, proteins, nutrients, hormones, enzymes, and wastes. Lymph contains many lymphocytes, other white blood cells, and some red blood cells. Lymph fluid moves slowly through the lymphatic network, with approximately three liters returning to the body's bloodstream every 24 hours (Marieb, 1998).

Summary

In summary, understanding alterations in ear, nose, throat, and head and neck anatomy and physiology is essential in determining the impact of head and neck cancer and its treatment. This knowledge is essential in planning appropriate nursing interventions and evaluating patient outcomes.

References

Alvord, L.S., & Farmer, B.L. (1997). Anatomy and orientation of the human external ear. *Journal of American Academy of Audiology, 8,* 383–390.

Andresen, H.G., Cyr, M.H., Guadagnini, J.P., Hickey, M.M., Higgins, T.S., Huntoon, M.B., et al. (1998). Normal anatomy and physiology. In L.L. Harris & M.B. Huntoon (Eds.), *Core curriculum for otorhinolaryngology and head-neck nursing* (pp. 33–61). New Smyrna Beach, FL: Society of Otorhinolaryngology and Head-Neck Nurses.

Bickley, L.S., & Szilagyi, P.G. (2003). *Bates' guide to physical examination and history taking* (8th ed.). Philadelphia: Lippincott Williams & Wilkins.

Duckert, L.G. (1998). Anatomy of the skull base, temporal bone, external ear, and middle ear. In C.W. Cummings, J.M. Frederickson, L.A. Harker, C.J. Krause, D.E. Schuller, & M.A. Richardson (Eds.), *Otolaryngology—head and neck surgery: Vol. 3* (3rd ed., pp. 2533–2546). St. Louis, MO: Mosby.

Graney, D.O., & Baker, S.R. (1998). Anatomy. In C.W. Cummings, J.M. Frederickson, L.A. Harker, C.J. Krause, D.E. Schuller, & M.A. Richardson (Eds.), *Otolaryngology—head and neck surgery: Vol. 2* (3rd ed., pp. 757–769). St. Louis, MO: Mosby.

Marieb, E.N. (1998). *Human anatomy and physiology* (4th ed.). Menlo Park, CA: Benjamin/Cummings Science Publishing.

McMinn, R.M.H., Hutchings, R.T., & Logan, B.M. (1994). *Color atlas of head and neck anatomy* (2nd ed.). London: Mosby-Wolfe.

Schwab, J., & Zenkel, M. (1998). Filtration of particles in the human nose. *Laryngoscope, 108,* 120–124.

Seeley, R.R., Stephens, T.D., & Tate, P. (1998). *Anatomy and physiology* (4th ed.). Boston: WBC/McGraw-Hill.

Shidnia, H., & Hornback, N.B. (1999). Radiation therapy of tumors of the salivary glands. In S.E. Thawley, W.R. Panje, J.G. Batsakis, & R.D. Lindberg (Eds.), *Comprehensive management of head and neck tumors: Vol. 2* (2nd ed., pp. 1182–1196). Philadelphia: W.B. Saunders.

Sigler, B.A., & Schuring, L.T. (1993). *Ear, nose, and throat disorders.* St. Louis, MO: Mosby.

CHAPTER 3

Pathophysiology

Margaret M. Hickey, RN, MSN, MS, OCN®, CORLN

Introduction

During the past 25 years, the process of what is required to turn a normal cell into a cancer cell has become more clear. Today, we know cancer is a group of diseases that results from genetic mutations that transform healthy cells into cancer cells. Genetic mutations can occur as a result of the effects of chemicals, viruses, radiation, and "mistakes" made each day in the course of duplicating DNA when a cell divides. Some individuals may inherit genetic mutations and, therefore, carry a higher lifetime risk of developing cancer because fewer subsequent changes in DNA are required to transform normal cells into cancer cells (National Cancer Institute [NCI], 1998).

Carcinogenesis

Carcinogenic theory suggests that cancer is the result of a series of genetic mutations. No one genetic alteration is enough to make a normal healthy cell a cancer cell. Cancer develops in a series of steps, with molecular changes progressing through preinvasive histologic changes to invasive disease. It is not yet fully understood how these genetic errors occur or why they are not corrected by the cell's efficient surveillance mechanisms. Initiating and promoting factors may be endogenous or exogenous. The number, type, and sequence of genetic errors required for initiation and promotion remain unknown for the majority of cancers (Foltz & Mahon, 2000).

Carcinogenesis occurs at the molecular level. The earliest events of this process, or initiation, begin in the genome. These may involve a point mutation in DNA, gene deletion, or chromosomal translocation resulting in gene rearrangement. These genetic alterations are not immediately responsible for morphologic changes (i.e., tissue structural changes). Cancer results after a progressive series of promoting events that incrementally increase the extent of deregulation within a cell line (see Figure 3-1). These events include a failure of DNA repair, activation of oncogenes, and loss of tumor suppressor function. The process interferes with apoptosis—the programmed death of abnormal or damaged cells—and a cell eventually results whose descendants continue to multiply without restraints (Giarelli, Jacobs, & Jenkins, 2002).

This "multi-hit" concept explains that more than one mutation needs to occur before a cancer will be evident. Initiation is the first step in this process in which the cell is originally altered so that it or its descendants are capable of behaving as cancer. These altered cells may alter apoptosis, cell product production, or cell function. Multiple factors may cause the initial malignant transformation at the genome level. Many cells are initiated through exposure to carcinogens. These carcinogens can be chemical, such as tobacco smoke or asbestos; physical, such as ionizing radiation; or biologic, such as viruses or bacteria. The body's complex DNA repair mechanism frequently repairs the damage, halting the progression of many initiated cells from developing into cancer (Foltz & Mahon, 2000).

For these genetically altered cells (initiated cells) to progress to cancer cells, a second series of events, or promotion, needs to occur. If the DNA repair is incomplete or new genetic errors are introduced during the repair processes and the initiated cell escapes the immune system, the abnormal cells proliferate. This process often is promoted by repeated exposure to carcinogens or other factors, and the tumor forms

---

Figure 3-1. Carcinogenic Sequence

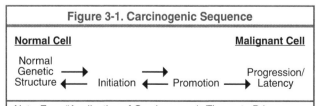

Note. From "Application of Carcinogenesis Theory to Primary Prevention," by A.T. Foltz and S.M. Mahon, 2000, *Oncology Nursing Forum, 27*(Suppl. 9), p. 6. Copyright 2000 by the Oncology Nursing Society. Reprinted with permission.

as the initiated cell is exposed to promoters. Once the cancer cell population fully develops, it continues to progress as the tumors enlarge and spread along a disease course (Foltz & Mahon, 2000; Giarelli et al., 2002).

Although in some tumor types, such as lung and colon cancer, the process of carcinogenesis has been well described, continued research is under way to understand this process in other tumors, including head and neck tumors. Continued interest is evident in the call for grant applications by the National Institute of Dental and Craniofacial Research (NIDCR) to foster basic research to decipher the molecular networks involved in the development of squamous cell carcinomas of the head and neck (NIDCR, 2003). There seems to be a relationship of genetic changes with the environment and behaviors, particularly alcohol consumption and/or smoking and tobacco use. These two factors are critical for patients with head and neck cancer, in whom tobacco use and alcohol abuse seem to have a synergistic, causal effect for squamous cell carcinomas of the head and neck.

Stages of Carcinogenesis

Initiation

Cancer begins with one or more genetic mutations resulting in unstable cells. Mutations that are unchecked start a cascade of further genetic events that can lead to uncontrolled cell growth and tumor formation (see Figure 3-2). Classes of genes involved in initiation are (a) oncogenes that accelerate cell growth, (b) mutated DNA mismatch-repair genes that fail to repair mistakes during cell division, and (c) mutated tumor suppressor genes that fail to stop cellular proliferation (Lea, Calzone, Masny, & Parry Bush, 2002).

An oncogene is a gene that when mutated or expressed at abnormally high levels, its protein products stimulate cellular division and viability by inhibiting apoptosis (Emory University Winship Cancer Institute, 2003). Prior to mutation, an oncogene often is called a proto-oncogene. Oncogenes are dominant; one defective allele can predispose the cell to tumor formation. If the cell has one normal gene (proto-oncogene) at a site and one mutated gene (the oncogene), the abnormal product takes control. Numerous oncogenes have been identified to date, including *ras, myc, ABL,* and *HER2.* No single oncogene can, by itself, cause cancer. It can, however, increase the rate of mitosis of the cell. Dividing cells are at increased risk for acquiring mutations, so a clone of an actively dividing cell is at risk for developing subclones with second, third, or more oncogenes. Once a cell loses all control over its mitosis, it is well on its way to developing into a cancer (Kimball, 2003).

As with many other diseases, both genetic and environmental factors are implicated in the development of cancer. Viral, chemical, and physical environmental factors can cause DNA mutations. These include physical factors, such as ionizing radiation; chemical factors, such as hydrocarbons, including those found in cigarette smoke; and specific tumor viruses—viruses with DNA genomes (e.g., papilloma, adenoviruses, herpes virus) and those with RNA genomes (retroviruses), such as HIV (Mellors, 1995). Some 15% of cases of head and neck cancer are linked to viral etiology (Joseph & Baibak, 2004). Epstein-Barr virus, a type of herpes virus

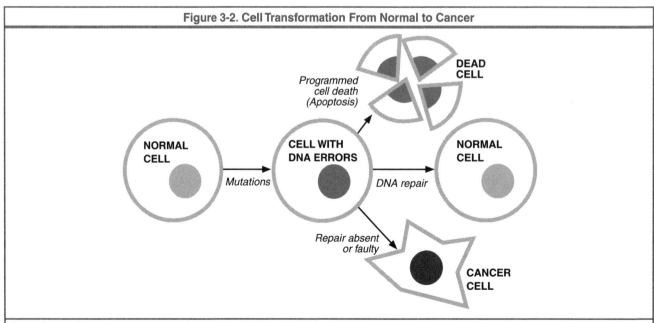

Figure 3-2. Cell Transformation From Normal to Cancer

NORMAL CELL

Mutations

CELL WITH DNA ERRORS

Programmed cell death (Apoptosis)

DEAD CELL

DNA repair

NORMAL CELL

Repair absent or faulty

CANCER CELL

Note. From *NCI Research Programs: Cancer Biology,* by National Cancer Institute, 1998, Bethesda, MD: Author. Retrieved November 27, 2003, from http://plan1998.cancer.gov/RESRCH.html

and the cause of infectious mononucleosis, is implicated in the development of nasopharyngeal carcinoma, and approximately 36% of those with oral cancer are infected with human papillomavirus-16 (Joseph & Baibak).

Failure to repair DNA produces a mutation. The human genome has been revealed to contain more than 100 genes whose products participate in DNA repair. Therefore, any gene whose product participates in DNA repair probably also can behave as an oncogene when mutated (Kimball, 2003; Mellors, 1995).

Cancer cells are engaged in uncontrolled mitosis. Some genes, known as tumor suppressor genes, whose protein products directly or indirectly inhibit cellular mitosis or lead to apoptosis, help to limit cellular proliferation. An example of a tumor suppressor gene is *p53*. The *p53* protein prevents a cell from completing the cell cycle if its DNA is not properly replicated in S phase. If the damage is minor, *p53* halts the cell cycle, preventing cell division until the damage is repaired. If the damage is major and cannot be repaired, *p53* triggers the cell to self-destruct through apoptosis. Mutations to tumor suppressor genes behave as recessive alleles. Tumor suppression will continue as long as the cell contains one normal allele. The tumor suppressor gene *p53* is key in protecting against cancer. More than half of all human cancers are known to have *p53* mutations and have no functioning *p53* protein (Kimball, 2003). Mutations of the *p53* gene are a common finding in patients with head and neck cancer. In squamous cell carcinoma, mutations in the *p53* gene correlate with alcohol and tobacco habits (Joseph & Baibak, 2004).

It may be years before cancer manifests. This is called the latency period. During this time, the tumor undergoes promotion. The body is unable to repair the genetic damage, and the altered cells elude the immune system. Further genetic changes occur, perhaps caused by exposure to carcinogens. The cells divide, and, over time, a malignancy develops. A latency period of 10 years or longer may elapse before the initial contact with the carcinogen and cancer cell initiation result in the appearance of the tumor (Mellors, 1995).

Initiation and promotion are two stages in the development of tumors. Chemical, physical, or biologic agents that irrevocably and genetically alter the cell genome result in initiation. Initiators cause genetic damage and need only a single exposure to start the cancer-forming process. Promoters may cause chemical or physical irritation, inflammation, and/or cellular growth when applied alone, but when applied after exposure to an initiator, they increase the rate of tumor formation and growth (Information Ventures, 1993).

Promotion

The mechanism of promotion is not well understood. It has been studied in animal models and was reported by T.J. Slaga in 1983. Promoters can amplify the development of a cancer in a number of ways. They may not be directly mutagenic or may only be weakly mutagenic; however, they can stimulate cell proliferation, allowing the initiated cancer cells to continue to propagate abnormally. Promotion at first may be reversible but later becomes irreversible. Another way in which promotion can occur is through inhibition of the body's natural defense, particularly the immune system. Lastly, promoters can alter the body's normal homeostasis, making it more favorable for tumor growth (Mellors, 1995; Slaga, 1983).

Progression

Progression, the third stage of neoplastic development, is separate from promotion. Progression, like initiation, involves molecular genetic changes; however, these changes are very different from the genetic changes of initiation (Malins, Polissar, & Gunselman, 1996; Mellors, 1995).

Four stages of tumor progression have been described for solid tumors, carcinomas, and sarcomas. Specific DNA mutations also have been identified in the sequence of progression from mild dysplasia to atypia to carcinoma in situ to invasive carcinoma. In patients with head and neck cancer, leukoplakia and erythroplakia are clinically identifiable lesions of the head and neck that may harbor invasive cancer or may undergo malignant transformation.

Hyperplasia is the earliest stage in which the altered cell divides in an uncontrolled manner, resulting in an excess of cells in a certain region. These cells continue to have a normal appearance; however, they are atypical because of the overpopulation (Emory University Winship Cancer Institute, 2003). An example of hyperplasia in a patient with a lesion of the head and neck is leukoplakia. *Leukoplakia* should be used only as a clinically descriptive term meaning the observer sees a white patch that does not rub off, the significance of which depends on the histologic findings. Leukoplakia results from chronic irritation of mucous membranes by carcinogens; this irritation stimulates the proliferation of white epithelia and connective tissue. Leukoplakia can range from hyperkeratosis associated with underlying epithelial hyperplasia to an actual early invasive carcinoma or may only represent a fungal infection, lichen planus, or other benign oral disease. In the absence of underlying dysplasia, leukoplakia rarely (< 5%) is associated with progression to malignancy (NCI, 2003a; Ridge, Glisson, Horwitz, & Meyers, 2004).

As cells continue to multiply uncontrolled, the risk of additional genetic alterations increases, and if tumor progression continues, *dysplasia* is the next stage. The cells and the tissue cannot yet be described as cancerous, but they no longer look normal. Dysplasia is characterized by cellular atypia, loss of normal maturation, and loss of normal epithelial stratification. It is graded as mild, moderate, or severe based on the degree of nuclear abnormality. In the transition from mild to severe dysplasia, nuclear abnormalities become more marked, mitoses become more apparent, and these changes involve increasing depth of epithelium. The likelihood of developing a carcinoma relates to the degrees of dysplasia. In cases where severe dysplasia is found in the head and neck, as many as 24% of patients may develop invasive squamous cell carcinoma (Ridge et al., 2004). *Erythroplakia* is a common finding in patients with head and neck cancer and is characterized by superficial, friable red patches adjacent to normal mucosa. It is commonly associated with underlying epithelial dysplasia and has a much greater potential for malignancy than leukoplakia. Carcinoma is found in nearly 40% of erythroplakia lesions (Ridge et al.).

Additional changes make the cells and tissues appear more abnormal, resulting in carcinoma in situ. It is unlike mild or moderate dysplasia, in which similar changes are seen but only a portion of the thickness of the epithelium is involved. *Carcinoma in situ* of the head and neck is characterized by the presence of dysplastic changes throughout the entire thickness of the epithelium with loss of normal maturation. These cells have an abnormally fast mitotic rate and bear little or no resemblance to normal cells. They may regress or become more primitive in their capabilities, often unable to complete normal functions. An example would be a liver cell that no longer makes liver-specific proteins. Cells of this type are said to be de-differentiated or anaplastic. Carcinoma in situ lesions often are described as preinvasive, as they are limited to one area. Carcinoma in situ is not reversible and is expected to become an invasive carcinoma if left untreated. These growths are considered to have the potential to become invasive and are treated as malignant growths. Tumors of this type often are curable by surgery because the abnormal cells are limited to one area. Once the dysplastic squamous cells move beyond the borders of the basement membrane (basal lamina), the lesion is referred to as invasive squamous cell carcinoma (Saunders & Wakely, n.d.). As the tumor cells continue to grow, they can invade surrounding tissues and/or spread (metastasize) outside of the local area. Benign tumors do not spread to tissues around them or to other parts of the body and are not cancerous. However, benign tumors still can cause serious health problems because they may put pressure on other organs and impair function. For example, meningioma, a common (usually benign) brain tumor, is slow growing but, given the limited space within the skull, can have serious consequences as a growth in the brain cavity, can have considerable morbidity, and may be fatal. Invasive cancers (malignant tumors) have the ability to invade surrounding tissues and/or metastasize through the vascular system or the lymph system to areas beyond the originating tissue. Malignant tumors can be life threatening.

Characteristics of Cancer Cells

Cancer cells are different from normal cells in that they are able to form a tumor and eventually metastasize to other parts of the body. When a normal cell is transformed to a cell capable of cancerous growth, a number of changes occur. Cancer cells acquire abilities that allow cellular proliferation despite the signals from the cells' environment. Normal cells will stop division in the presence of genetic (DNA) damage; cancer cells will continue to divide. The results are "daughter" cells that contain abnormal DNA. These daughter cells progressively evolve to become even more abnormal. Normal cells require growth signals before they can move from a resting state into an active proliferative state. Cancer cells will proliferate in the absence of these growth signals. Noticeable changes also occur in the physical properties of the cell. Alterations in the cytoskeleton of the cell affect cellular adhesion and motility. Cancer cells do not exhibit contact inhibition, one of the cellular growth inhibitory signals. Normal cellular growth is checked as cells respond to contact inhibition and cease to divide when they sense they are being "crowded" by other cells. The reduction of cell-to-cell and cell-to-extracellular matrix adhesion allows large masses of cells to form. Without contact inhibition, tumor cells continue to divide even when surrounded by other cells, the cells continue to "pile up," and a tumor is formed. Normal cellular adhesion prevents normal cells from moving. The cytoskeletal alterations affecting cellular adhesion allow the cancer cells to move about. Cancer cells must be able to move and migrate in order to spread.

The shape and organization of the nuclei of cancer cells may be markedly different from the nuclei of normal cells of the same origin. These changes are useful in diagnosing and staging tumors. Cancer cells often secrete enzymes that digest the barriers to migration and enable invasion into neighboring tissues, aiding in the spread of the tumor (Emory University Winship Cancer Institute, 2003).

Changes in Cancer Cells

The changes seen in individual cells are mirrored by the behavior of the tumors. For a tumor to grow and invade neighboring tissues, several major changes must occur. Hanahan and Weinberg (2000) have detailed a model of cancer growth and metastasis. Cancer cells and tumors must acquire a specific set of abilities. These include (a) growth signal autonomy, (b) insensitivity to antigrowth signals, (c) resistance to apoptosis, (d) limitless replicative potential, (e) sustained angiogenesis, and (f) tissue invasion and metastasis.

Growth Signal Autonomy

Normal cells will not reproduce unless they receive external signals that cause the cells to enter into the cell cycle. Cancer cells are able to proliferate by entering the cell cycle independent of external signaling. Three processes are described to explain how cancer cells acquire growth signal autonomy. First, many cancer cells acquire the ability to synthesize growth factors to which they are responsive, eliminating dependence on other cells within the tissue. Second, cell surface receptors transmit growth signals into the cell interior. Receptor overexpression may cause the cancer cell to become hyperresponsive to low levels of growth factor that would not normally trigger proliferation. Third, cancer cells can switch the types of extracellular matrix receptors they express to favor ones that transmit progrowth signals. One cell that divides without proper growth signals results in a population of daughter cells that also divide autonomously of growth signals.

Insensitivity to Antigrowth Signals

The division of normal cells is restricted through multiple antigrowth signals. These signals include both soluble growth inhibitors and inhibitors fixed in the extracellular matrix and on the surfaces of nearby cells. Two distinct mechanisms exist to block cells from entering the cell cycle and dividing. One forces cells out of active proliferation into the resting (G0) state until some future extracellular growth signal permits it to reenter the cell cycle. A second mechanism occurs in which cells permanently relinquish their ability to divide by entering a postmitotic state. This state usually is associated with cellular differentiation when a precursor cell continues to differentiate, acquiring its final functional capabilities. Cancer cells must evade these antigrowth signals specifically through disruptions of the pathways that govern the transit of the cell through the cell cycle. At the molecular level, many, if not all, of the antiproliferative signals are channeled through the retinoblastoma protein (pRb) and its two relatives p1-7 and p130. To illustrate, disruption of the pRb pathway releases E2F transcription factors, allowing cell proliferation and making cells insensitive to antigrowth factors that normally operate along this pathway. Human tumors have been found to disrupt the pRb pathway in a variety of ways, thus creating insensitivity to antigrowth signals (Hanahan & Weinberg, 2000).

Normal cells will stop dividing when they are in contact with neighboring cells. The cell-to-cell contact immobilizes cells and sends signals to the dividing cells to stop them from dividing. Cancer cells undergo cytoskeletal changes rendering them nonresponsive to this normal cellular growth brake.

Resistance to Apoptosis

In normal tissue, a balance between new cells is created through cell division and the loss of cells through cell death. A process termed *apoptosis,* or programmed cell death, eliminates cells that become damaged. Apoptosis is a precisely choreographed series of steps during which (a) the cellular membranes are disrupted, (b) the cytoplasmic and nuclear skeletons are broken down, (c) the cytosol is extruded, (d) the chromosomes are degraded, (e) the cell is fragmented, and (f) the debris is consumed by nearby phagocytic cells. This process is a normal and necessary safeguard that allows for the identification and elimination of mutated or damaged cells.

The ability of tumor cell populations to grow is a result of not only the rate of cell proliferation but also the rate of cell death. Increasing evidence suggests resistance to apoptosis is a hallmark of most, if not all, types of cancers. Apoptotic machinery can be divided into two components—sensors and effectors. Sensors monitor the extracellular and intracellular environment for conditions of normality or abnormality that indicate whether a cell will live or die. Extracellular sensors are maintained for most cells by the cellular matrix and cell-to-cell adherence-based survival signals. Intracellular sensors monitor the cell and activate the "death pathway" in response to detection of abnormalities including DNA damage, signaling imbalance provoked by oncogenes, or hypoxia.

When activated, the intracellular and extracellular sensors send signals to regulate the effectors of apoptotic death. The signals that prompt apoptosis converge on the mitochondrion, which responds by releasing cytochrome C, a potent catalyst of apoptosis. The ultimate effectors of apoptosis include an array of intracellular proteases, termed *capsases.* These capsases trigger activation of a dozen or more effector capsases that execute the death program. Cancer cells can acquire resistance to apoptosis through a variety of strategies. The most common is the loss of a pro-apoptotic regulator involving mutation of the *p53* tumor suppressor gene (Hanahan & Weinberg, 2000).

Limitless Replicative Potential

In theory, deregulation of cellular proliferation through growth signal autonomy, insensitivity to antigrowth signals, and resistance to apoptosis should suffice in leading to the vast cell populations that create tumors. However, this disruption of cell-to-cell signaling alone does not guarantee expansive tumor growth. Many, if not all, mammalian cells carry an intrinsic cell autonomous program that limits cell multiplication. This appears to operate independently of the pathways previously described. It, too, must be disrupted for cancer cells to expand to an overt and potentially life-threatening tumor. Although normal cells only can divide a finite number of times before stopping cell division and dying, cancer cells have the ability to divide endlessly without appearing to "age," as seen in noncancer cells. In many cancers, this is because of the activation of an enzyme, telomerase. Telomerase functions to maintain the integrity of the chromosomes during cell division (Hanahan & Weinberg, 2000).

Sustained Angiogenesis

Oxygen and nutrients supplied by the vasculature are crucial for cell function and survival. During organ formation, blood supply is ensured through coordinated growth of new blood vessels. In normal cellular growth, once a tissue is formed, the growth of new blood vessels, or angiogenesis, is transitory and carefully regulated.

The development of blood vessels is an essential step in the growth and metastasis of a tumor. Tumors can grow up to 1–2 mm without neovascularization, but they cannot metastasize and grow above this size without new blood vessel growth (Marshall, 2004). For a tumor to progress in size, it must develop angiogenic ability. Tumor cells or adjacent cells produce angiogenic growth factors to stimulate the formation of new blood vessels. Angiogenic activators include vascular endothelial growth factor, basic fibroblast growth factor, and transforming growth factors. Without angiogenesis, tumor cell proliferation is inhibited because it is matched or exceeded by apoptosis. The ability to induce or sustain angiogenesis seems to be acquired in a discrete step during tumor development when tumor cell proliferation exceeds apoptosis (Hanahan & Weinberg, 2000; Marshall).

Tissue Invasion and Metastasis

Sooner or later during the development of most cancers, primary tumor masses can move through the blood or lymphatic systems or through direct contact to another location. When a cancer cell has moved, it may divide and form a tumor at the new site (metastasis). Metastatic tumors often interfere with organ function and lead to the morbidity and mortality seen with cancer. The majority of cancer deaths are a result of metastasis of the cancer to sites distant from the primary site (Emory University Winship Cancer Institute, 2003).

Invasion and metastasis are closely allied processes. For cells to move through the body, they must first "climb" over and around neighboring cells. They do this by rearranging their cytoskeleton and attaching to the other cells and the extracellular matrix via proteins on the outside of their plasma membrane. Cells migrate or move until stopped by the basal lamina or basement membrane. To cross this membrane, cancer cells secrete enzymes called matrix metalloproteases. These enzymes degrade the proteins in the basal lamina and allow continued migration and invasion into adjacent tissues as well as to distant locations via adjacent blood vessels or lymphatic vessels (Emory University Winship Cancer Institute, 2003).

Metastasis, or spread outside of the primary site, can occur through invasion of the cancer cells by direct contact with other organs or via cancer cell migration into the lymphatic system or vasculature. The lymphatic system is an extensive network with lymphatic flow throughout the body, much like the circulatory system. Cancer cells move into the lymphatic system and then can deposit nearby or distantly from the primary tumor site. The tumor cells can be found in the lymph nodes. This helps to identify the extent of metastatic disease and tumor staging (Emory University Winship Cancer Institute, 2003).

Hematogenous metastasis, or the spread of cancer cells through the circulatory system, results from the cells migrating among the blood vessel epithelial cells. Once in the blood, the cancer cell embolism is carried through the circulatory system until it finds a suitable location in which to settle and reenter the tissues (see Figure 3-3) (Mellors, 1995).

Hematogenous and lymphatic metastases result in the cancer cells settling in a distant location and forming a new tumor. The tumor cells that have metastasized to a distant

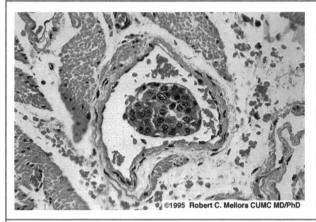

Figure 3-3. Tumor Embolism in Esophageal Blood Vessel

©1995 Robert C. Mellors CUMC MD/PhD

Note. Copyright 1995 by Robert C. Mellors, MD, PhD. Used with permission.

location retain the characteristics they had when they were in their original location.

Behavior of cancers of the head and neck depends on the site of origin. Each anatomic site predisposes the metastatic pattern and prognosis. Regional invasion usually reaches beyond the anatomic limits of the primary site deep into the neighboring structures and along tissue planes. The perineural route is also an important pathway for metastasis of head and neck cancers. Intracranial spread can occur along the peripheral branches of the cranial nerves.

Regional and distant metastases are most likely caused by invasion of the lymphatic system because the head and neck region is rich in lymphatic drainage. Extension of the cancer cells into the regional lymph nodes is more likely to occur with larger lesions (2–4 cm) and lesions found in sites with abundant lymphatic drainage (Baylor College of Medicine, 1996). If the primary site is near the midline, contralateral or bilateral metastases should be anticipated. Important prognostic factors in head and neck cancer include tumor size, lymph node spread, and distant metastasis. With lymph node spread, the presence of extracapsular nodal involvement of the tumor is an important negative prognostic factor in head and neck cancer (Ridge et al., 2004). The more poorly differentiated (more aggressive) tumors tend to metastasize early to regional lymph nodes and beyond (Harris, 2000). Stennert et al. (2003) published their experience in a retrospective review of salivary gland tumors reporting the frequency of lymph node metastasis in head and neck lesions and the significance of nodal status to overall and disease-free survival.

Distant metastasis is not commonly seen in squamous cell carcinoma of the head and neck. In the past, it was believed that head and neck tumors rarely metastasized beyond the lymph nodes. However, as local regional control improves and individuals are living longer, the incidence of hematogenous metastases increases, with the lung as the most common site of metastasis. Hematogenous metastasis is less common than lymphatic metastasis in head and neck cancer. It usually is seen in late-stage disease or in more aggressive tumors (Harris, 2000).

Histology

Squamous cell (epidermoid) carcinomas comprise 90%–95% of head and neck cancers; less common histologies for tumors of the mucosal areas are adenocarcinoma and lymphoepithelioma. Tumors of the glandular tissue of the head and neck differ in histology from those arising in the upper airways and digestive tract. Parotid gland tumors are the most common of the salivary gland tumors and are typically benign (75%–80%). However, 35%–40% of the submandibular tumors and 90% of sublingual tumors are malignant. The most common benign tumor type is pleomorphic adenoma. Malignant tumors include mucoepidermoid carcinoma, adenoid cystic carcinoma, acinic cell carcinoma, and squamous cell carcinoma (Baylor College of Medicine, 1996; NCI, 2003c).

Head and neck cancers encompass a diverse group of tumors that are frequently aggressive in their biologic behavior. Patients with head and neck cancer often develop a second primary tumor. The incidence of second cancers increases more dramatically in patients who continue to smoke. Overall, second primary tumors occur at an annual rate of 3%–7%, and 50%–75% of such new cancers occur in the upper aerodigestive tract or lung (Ridge et al., 2004).

Squamous Cell Carcinoma

Squamous cell carcinoma is a malignant neoplasm of epithelial origin that develops from the epithelial cells lining the surface of the upper airway and aerodigestive tract. Squamous cell carcinomas are mucosal lesions and usually are visible at the surface; they rarely develop beneath an intact-appearing mucosa. *Squamous cell carcinoma* can be used interchangeably with *epidermoid carcinoma,* although the latter is less commonly used.

Morphologic appearance of squamous cell carcinoma is variable, and these tumors may appear as plaques, nodules, or wart-like growths. These lesions may be scaly or ulcerated, white, red, or brown (Joseph & Baibak, 2004). Invasive squamous cell carcinoma initially infiltrates the subepithelial fibrous tissue. The tissue invaded in later stages depends on the site of the tumor. Muscle invasion is a common feature, with bone and/or cartilage invasion usually seen as a late phenomenon. Perineural spread along the nerve sheaths and/or perivascular spread can be seen at all head and neck sites. Locoregional spread results from invasion of the lymphatic capillaries, with subsequent metastasis to cervical lymph nodes.

Hematogenous metastasis is uncommon, but if it occurs, the usual site of metastasis is the lung (Hermans, 2001).

Squamous cell carcinoma may arise from dysplastic epithelium or may arise without dysplastic changes being noted. The hallmark of invasive squamous cell carcinoma (especially in low-grade lesions) is the presence of keratin or "keratin pearls" on histologic evaluation. Keratin is the end product of squamous cell degeneration and normally is found in skin and some squamous mucosa, excluding the larynx. Keratin pearls are eosinophilic and roundish and have a thin membrane. For reasons unknown, keratin pearls are not found in carcinoma in situ (Saunders & Wakely, n.d.).

Microscopically, the nuclei of malignant squamous cells are rich with DNA and will stain dark (hyperchromatic). The nucleus is likely to be large in proportion to the cytoplasm; the nuclear-cytoplasmic ratio may be 1:1 instead of the normal 1:4 or 1:6. The nuclear shape may be variable. Mitotic figures may be numerous and often are abnormal in appearance, with large spindles in one area and shrunken spindles in others. Tumor giant cells may be present with a single huge polymorphic nucleus and others with two or more nuclei. The orientation of tumor cells to one another is erratic compared to the orderly arrangement seen in normal tissue. Large masses of cells are seen, and "fingers" of tumor cells may be invading adjacent normal tissue (Saunders & Wakely, n.d.).

Verrucous Carcinoma

Verrucous carcinoma is a rare variant of well-differentiated (low-grade) squamous cell carcinoma that was first described by Lauren Ackerman in 1948. It is an uncommon variant in the United States usually occurring in white males older than 55–65 years of age. It typically appears at sites of chronic irritation and inflammation. Human papillomavirus may be a risk factor for development of verrucous carcinoma as well as association with chewing tobacco, snuff, and betel nuts. It most frequently is found in the oral cavity. Human papilloma virus-16 frequently has been identified in these lesions. Verrucous carcinoma is characterized as an exophytic, gray, bulky lesion with a papillomatous and fungating appearance. It is sometimes described as a well-differentiated papillomatous tumor because of the papillomatous character of the lesion. This well-differentiated squamous carcinoma is much less invasive and rarely metastasizes. In the rare instance that metastasis occurs, it is usually to regional lymph nodes. However, these tumors can become problematic because they may grow to be quite large and potentially may lead to upper airway obstruction (Ali & Zeina, 2004; Callender, 1991).

Microscopically, the cells show none of the mitoses or dysplastic features usually seen with squamous carcinoma. The surface shows characteristic "church-spire" formations because of extensive keratinization (Saunders & Wakely, n.d.). This lesion is composed of highly differentiated squamous cells, is broadly based, and has a large blunt-ended network of ridges with an intact basement membrane. An inflammatory reaction also often is present in the stroma composed of lymphocytes and plasma cells (Callender, 1991).

Treatment consists of surgery or radiation and is considered to be curative if the entire lesion is excised. Overall, surgery is the most effective therapy (Ali & Zeina, 2004). Occasionally, the lesions may change to frankly invasive carcinoma (Saunders & Wakely, n.d.).

Lymphoepithelioma

Another variant of squamous carcinoma that is sometimes referred to as anaplastic squamous cell carcinoma is lymphoepithelioma. Lymphoepithelioma also is known as lymphoepithelial carcinoma, Schmincke tumor, or Regaud tumor. It is extremely rare, with the highest frequency found among young adults of East Asian/Eskimo origin (Dorland, 2003; SEER Training, n.d.).

Lymphoepithelioma is a carcinoma with a lymphoid stroma predominantly occurring in the nasopharynx, parotid gland, or tonsils. It also may be described as an undifferentiated carcinoma of nasopharyngeal type. It occurs at sites with lymphoid aggregates within the submucosa, namely Waldeyer ring. Infection with the Epstein-Barr virus seems to play an important etiologic role (Hermans, 2001; Stanley, Weiland, DeSanto, & Neel, 1985).

Microscopically, lymphoepithelioma is a pleomorphic, poorly differentiated (transitional cell) carcinoma arising from the epithelium that overlies the lymphoid tissue of the nasopharynx or tonsil. It is composed of irregular sheets, or small groups, of neoplastic epithelial cells (squamous or undifferentiated), with a slight to moderate amount of fibrous stroma containing numerous lymphocytes. It metastasizes early to cervical lymph nodes (Dorland, 2003).

Spindle Cell Carcinoma

Spindle cell carcinoma is a rare and unusual form of poorly differentiated squamous cell carcinoma with elongated or spindled epithelial cells that resemble sarcoma spindle cell morphology. It may be invasive or in situ (Saunders & Wakely, n.d.). It also is referred to as sarcomatoid squamous cell carcinoma and polypoid squamous cell carcinoma (Oral and Maxillofacial Pathology List, n.d.).

Microscopically, the presence of keratin and DNA content in the spindle cell population supports the neoplastic epithelial origin of these neoplasms. The overall tumor behavior and surgical therapy appeared to be comparable with those of squamous cell carcinomas at a similar stage (Olsen, Lewis, & Suman, 1997).

There seem to be no specific risk factors such as smoking associated with spindle cell carcinoma. When lymph node metastases are found, the cell type may represent either the spindle cell or squamous cell component. Surgery is the most effective therapy; however, overall prognosis is poor (Saunders & Wakely, n.d.).

Histologic Grading

Squamous cell carcinoma is graded on a scale of I–IV. Grading is done according to the degree the cells have departed histologically from their normal appearance. Lower grade lesions are better differentiated and closely resemble normal epithelium. Higher grade lesions, III or IV, are significantly deviated from normal cells, and with a grade IV lesion, it may be difficult to determine if the origin is from squamous epithelium. The terms *high grade, anaplastic,* or *poorly differentiated* are used. Individual pathologists' experiences and criteria will account for occasional differences in grading the same specimen (Saunders & Wakely, n.d.). Tumor grading is recommended using Broder's classification of tumor grade (G) (NCI, 2003a).

- G1—well-differentiated
- G2—moderately differentiated
- G3—poorly differentiated
- G4—undifferentiated

In general, the more poorly differentiated a lesion, the higher the incidence of regional metastases and poorer the prognosis. No statistically significant correlation between tumor grade and clinical behavior of the cancer has been shown. Features that predict aggressive behavior include perineural spread, lymphatic invasion, and tumor extension beyond the lymph node capsule (NCI, 2003b).

Salivary Gland Tumors

Salivary gland neoplasms are histologically diverse. These neoplasms include benign and malignant tumors. Grading of salivary gland tumors is used primarily for mucoepidermoid carcinoma; adenocarcinoma, not otherwise specified (NOS); adenoid cystic carcinoma; and squamous cell carcinoma. NCI (2003c) listed in its PDQ® treatment guide for healthcare professionals salivary gland carcinomas and the appropriate category according to histologic grade (see Figure 3-4).

Adenoid Cystic Carcinoma

Adenoid cystic carcinoma (formerly known as cylindroma) is a slow-growing but aggressive neoplasm with a remarkable ability to recur. It is a very lethal type of tumor, even when treated early (Baylor College of Medicine, 1996). This neoplasm usually presents as a slow-growing swelling in the preauricular or submandibular region. Pain and facial paralysis develop frequently during the course of the disease, a result of the high incidence of perineural invasion. Regardless of histologic grade, adenoid cystic carcinomas have an unusually slow biologic growth, a protracted course, and, ultimately, a poor outcome. The 10-year survival rate is reported to be less than 50% for all grades (NCI, 2003c). These carcinomas typically recur, and late distant metastasis occurs with patients dying of pulmonary metastasis. Clinical stage may be a better prognostic indicator than histologic grade. In a retrospective review of 92 cases, a tumor size greater than

---

Figure 3-4. Categories for Salivary Gland Carcinomas by Grade

Low grade
- Acinic cell carcinoma
- Basal cell adenocarcinoma
- Clear cell carcinoma
- Cystadenocarcinoma
- Epithelial-myoepithelial carcinoma
- Mucinous adenocarcinoma
- Polymorphous low-grade adenocarcinoma

Low grade, intermediate grade, and high grade
- Adenocarcinoma, not otherwise specified
- Mucoepidermoid carcinoma
- Squamous cell carcinoma

Intermediate grade and high grade
- Myoepithelial carcinoma

High grade
- Anaplastic small cell carcinoma
- Carcinosarcoma
- Large cell undifferentiated carcinoma
- Small cell undifferentiated carcinoma
- Salivary duct carcinoma

Note. Based on information from National Cancer Institute, 2003c.

---

4 cm was associated with an unfavorable clinical course in all cases (NCI, 2003c).

This malignant tumor is poorly encapsulated, and although it seems to be well defined within the gland, there is usually infiltration of the surrounding tissue. Morphologically, three growth patterns have been described: cribriform (classic), tubular, and solid (basaloid). The tumors are categorized according to the predominant pattern. The cribriform pattern shows epithelial cell nests forming a cylindrical pattern and giving it the classic "Swiss cheese" appearance. The tubular pattern is defined as such because of the tubular structures that are lined by stratified cuboidal epithelium. The solid pattern shows solid groups of cuboidal cells. The cribriform pattern is the most common, whereas the solid pattern is the least common. Solid adenoid cystic carcinoma is a high-grade lesion with reported recurrence rates of up to 100%, compared with 50%–80% for the tubular and cribriform variants (NCI, 2003c; Saunders & Wakely, n.d.).

Mucoepidermoid Carcinoma

Mucoepidermoid carcinoma is the most common malignant salivary gland neoplasm in both adults and children. Usually, they grow slowly and present as painless masses. They are poorly encapsulated or unencapsulated and easily infiltrate surrounding tissue. A wide range of biologic behavior may be seen. The majority of these tumors do not metastasize;

however, if metastasis occurs, it is to the regional nodes, bone, lung, and brain. Patients with well-differentiated tumors have a 90% five-year survival rate, whereas those with poorly differentiated tumors may have only a 20% five-year survival rate (Saunders & Wakely, n.d.). Treatment usually is surgical, with adjuvant radiation if needed (Saunders & Wakely).

This malignant epithelial tumor is composed of mucoid and epidermoid squamous cells. The mucoid cells are large with distinct borders and have a foamy cytoplasm that stains with mucin. The epidermoid squamous cells may show large nuclei with prominent nucleoli and an eosinophilic cytoplasm. The squamous cells are arranged in nests or solid areas in conjunction with mucoid cells. There may be some keratin deposits, but usually no large pearls as in squamous carcinoma. In addition to mucous and epidermal cells, there are "intermediate" cells, which are round to oval and basaloid with scant pink cytoplasm (Saunders & Wakely, n.d.).

Microscopic grading of mucoepidermoid carcinoma helps to determine prognosis. Mucous cells and cysts are prominent in low-grade tumors with minimal dysplastic cells. High-grade lesions are more squamous than mucinous and have significant pleomorphism and mitotic activity (Saunders & Wakely, n.d.).

Mucoepidermoid carcinomas are graded as low, intermediate, and high. NCI (2003c) provided the following grading parameters with assigned point values.
- Intracystic component (+2)
- Neural invasion present (+2)
- Necrosis present (+3)
- Mitosis (4 or more per 10 high power fields) (+3)
- Anaplasia present (+4)

Total point scores are 0–4 for low grade, 5–6 for intermediate, and 7–14 for high grade.

Adenocarcinoma

Adenocarcinoma is a malignant neoplasm with a microscopic glandular growth pattern. These tumors are particularly common in the head and neck, especially in tumors of the salivary glands. There are approximately 20 specific types of malignant epithelial salivary gland tumors and tumors from other sites. Clinically, patients typically present with a slowly enlarging mass in the parotid region. Pain related to the tendency for perineural invasion is a symptom in more than one-third of patients (Saunders & Wakely, n.d.).

Acinic Cell Carcinoma

Acinic cell carcinoma (also known as acinic cell adenocarcinoma) is a low-grade malignant epithelial neoplasm in which the cells express acinar differentiation. The term *acinic cell carcinoma* is used because of the differentiation toward serous acinar cells as opposed to mucous acinar cells (NCI, 2003c). The largest series of salivary tumors to date was reported in the Armed Forces Institute of Pathology (AFIP) salivary gland registry. AFIP identified acinic cell carcinoma as the third most common malignancy of salivary glands. Seventeen percent of primary malignant salivary gland tumors and approximately 6% of all salivary gland neoplasms were acinic cell carcinoma. Most of these (86%) occurred in the parotid gland. Women were affected more than men, and the median age at diagnosis was 52 years old (Hoffman, Karnell, Robinson, Pinkston, & Menck, 1999).

Staging is a better predictor of outcome than histologic grade. In a retrospective review of 90 cases at the Mayo Clinic, poor prognostic features included pain or fixation; gross invasion; and microscopic features of desmoplasia, atypia, or increased mitotic activity. Neither morphologic pattern nor cell composition was a predictive feature (Lewis, Olsen, & Weiland, 1991).

Polymorphous Low-Grade Adenocarcinoma

Polymorphous low-grade adenocarcinoma (PLGA) is a malignant epithelial tumor that is limited to the minor salivary gland sites. A bland, uniform nucleus and diverse architecture that infiltrates, particularly with perineural invasion, characterize these lesions. This neoplasm can be benign or malignant. It most commonly occurs in the mucosa of the soft or hard palate. The average age at diagnosis is 59, and it is twice as common in women as in men (NCI, 2003c).

PLGA typically presents as a firm, nontender swelling and usually runs a moderately indolent course. Because of the unpredictable behavior of the tumor, some investigators consider the qualifying term "low-grade" to be misleading and instead prefer the term "polymorphous adenocarcinoma" (Speight & Barrett, 2002).

Adenocarcinoma, Not Otherwise Specified

The term *adenocarcinoma, NOS,* is used for a subset of adenocarcinoma neoplasms that do not easily fit into the defined tumor subtypes. Approximately 40% occur in the major salivary glands and 60% in the minor glands. The mean patient age at diagnosis is 58 years (NCI, 2003c).

Adenocarcinoma, NOS, is a salivary gland carcinoma that presents a glandular growth pattern microscopically. The borders tend to be irregular, and there may be extension outside of the gland as found in other adenocarcinomas. Histologic diagnosis is one of exclusion more than inclusion. This tumor is graded according to the degree of differentiation, a manner similar to other salivary lesions. Tumor grades include low, intermediate, and high. Low-grade tumors may be well circumscribed with focal infiltration and contain well-formed duct-like structures with bland features and few mitoses. High-grade tumors also show glandular differentiation but with more solid areas of tumor growth, more mitoses, and greater nuclear variability. Tumor giant cells also may be present (Saunders & Wakely, n.d.).

Rare Adenocarcinomas

The glandular tissue of the salivary glands, both major and minor, lends itself to a number of rare adenocarcinomas. Because these pathologies are extremely rare, they will not be discussed, but a listing is provided. NCI (2003c) provided the following list.

- Basal cell adenocarcinoma
- Clear cell carcinoma
- Cystadenocarcinoma
- Sebaceous adenocarcinoma
- Sebaceous lymphadenocarcinoma
- Oncocytic carcinoma
- Salivary duct carcinoma
- Mucinous adenocarcinoma

Malignant Mixed Tumors

Malignant mixed tumors include three distinct entities: carcinoma ex pleomorphic adenoma, carcinosarcoma, and metastasizing mixed tumor. Most salivary neoplasms are carcinoma ex pleomorphic adenoma. Carcinosarcoma (true malignant mixed tumor) and metastasizing mixed tumor are extremely rare.

Carcinoma Ex Pleomorphic Adenoma

Carcinoma ex pleomorphic adenoma (also known as carcinoma ex mixed tumor) is a carcinoma showing evidence of arising from or in a benign pleomorphic adenoma. Diagnosis requires the identification of benign tumor in the tissue sample. The AFIP database reports that carcinoma ex pleomorphic adenoma comprises 4.6% of all malignant salivary gland tumors. The tumor occurs most commonly in the major salivary glands (Ellis & Auclair, 1996). Presentation is commonly a painless mass with facial paralysis. Tumor stage, histologic grade, and degree of invasion are important prognostic factors. Depending on the series cited, survival times vary significantly: 25%–65% at 5 years, 24%–50% at 10 years, 10%–35% at 15 years, and 0%–38% at 20 years (NCI, 2003c).

Carcinosarcoma

Carcinosarcoma (also known as true malignant mixed tumor) is an extremely rare malignant salivary gland neoplasm that contains both carcinoma and sarcoma components. Most of these tumors occur in the major salivary glands and present with swelling, pain, nerve palsy, and ulceration. Carcinosarcoma is an aggressive high-grade malignancy (NCI, 2003c).

Metastasizing Mixed Tumor

Metastasizing mixed tumor is a very rare histologically benign salivary gland neoplasm that unexplainably metastasizes. Most of them occur in the major salivary glands following a single well-defined primary mass. Often, a long interval occurs between the diagnosis of the primary tumor and the metastases. The histologic features are those seen in pleomorphic adenoma (NCI, 2003c).

Rare Carcinomas

The remaining salivary gland carcinomas are extremely rare and will not be discussed in any length but are only included in the following listing (NCI, 2003c).

- Primary squamous cell carcinoma
- Epithelial-myoepithelial carcinoma
- Anaplastic small cell carcinoma
- Undifferentiated carcinoma
- Small cell undifferentiated carcinoma (extrapulmonary oat cell carcinoma)
- Large cell undifferentiated carcinoma
- Myoepithelial carcinoma
- Adenosquamous carcinoma

Summary

Cancer is a general term for a group of diseases resulting from genetic cellular changes causing abnormal and uncontrolled cellular division, interfering with apoptosis, and altering the normal appearance and function of cells. As more is learned about the genetic code and cellular processes, a greater understanding of carcinogenesis is unfolding.

Cancers of the head and neck will account for almost 3% of the new cancer cases diagnosed in 2005 and nearly 2% of the deaths (American Cancer Society [ACS], 2005). ACS estimated that 20,780 cases of oral cancer, 8,590 pharynx cancers, and 9,880 cancers of the larynx will be diagnosed in 2005, resulting in more than 11,000 deaths. Cancers of the head and neck can be divided into sites and subsites, depending on the area in which the tumor originated. The most common sites for head and neck cancer include tumors of the oral cavity, salivary glands, paranasal sinuses, nasal cavity, pharynx, larynx, lymph nodes, and thyroid gland.

The epidemiology, natural history, and treatment approach are dependent on the tumor anatomic site. Squamous cell carcinoma is the most common pathology and accounts for more than 90% of the head and neck tumors. Head and neck cancers frequently are aggressive, and, unfortunately, most patients with head and neck cancer have metastatic disease at the time of diagnosis (43% nodal involvement and 10% distant metastasis). Patients with head and neck cancer often develop a second primary lesion, usually of the upper aerodigestive tract or lung, at an annual rate of 3%–7% (Ridge et al., 2004). Lifestyle modification is key to a patient's response to therapy as well as reducing the chance of a secondary malignancy. If a patient with a single cancer continues to smoke and use alcohol, the cure rate for the initial cancer regardless of treatment modality is diminished. Also, the risk of second primary tumors increases in up to 25% of patients whose initial lesion was controlled (NCI, 2004).

As more is learned about carcinogenesis and the natural history of head and neck cancer, there is potential to improve both curative and preventive treatments. Preventive measures include tobacco cessation programs and focus on other lifestyle modifications, such as elimination or reduction of alcohol use. Additionally, trials have focused on reducing the occurrence of second primaries. Isotretinoin (13-cis-retinoic acid) has been studied. Although Hong et al. (1990) reported that daily treatment with moderate doses of isotretinoin for one year could significantly reduce the incidence of second tumors, it did not result in any survival advantage. These findings were not supported in two randomized trials completed by the Italian Head and Neck Chemoprevention Study Group and the Southwest Oncology Group (Khuri et al., 2003; Toma et al., 2004).

Treatment measures also are being developed using what has been learned with the improved understanding of the role of tumor suppressor *p53* mutations in head and neck cancer. A potential new therapeutic agent, Advexin® (Introgen Therapeutics, Austin, TX), induces the expression of the tumor suppressor *p53* protein in very high concentrations in cancer tissue to selectively kill cancer cells. In December 2004, Introgen Therapeutics (2004) submitted a request to the U.S. Food and Drug Administration for approval of Advexin.

Understanding of the pathophysiology of head and neck cancer is key in laying the foundation to the development of future therapies and provides continued hope in the battle against cancers of the head and neck.

References

Ackerman, L.V. (1948). Verrucous carcinoma of the oral cavity. *Surgery, 23,* 670–678.

Ali, M., & Zeina, B. (2004, October). *Verrucous carcinoma. Treatment.* Retrieved November 5, 2004, from http://www.emedicine.com/derm/topic452.htm#section~treatment

American Cancer Society. (2005). *Cancer facts and figures, 2005.* Atlanta, GA: Author. Retrieved February 21, 2005, from http://www.cancer.org

Baylor College of Medicine. (1996). *Head and neck tumors.* Retrieved November 27, 2003, from http://www.bcm.tmc.edu/oto/studs/hnt.html

Callender, T.A. (1991, September). *Verrucous carcinoma of the head and neck. Grand Rounds Archives.* Retrieved December 29, 2003, from http://www.bcm.tmc.edu/oto/grand/92891.html

Dorland, W.A. (2003). *Dorland's illustrated medical dictionary* (30th ed.). St. Louis, MO: Elsevier.

Ellis, G.L., & Auclair, P.L. (1996). Tumors of the salivary glands. In *AFIP atlas of tumor pathology* (3rd ed., pp. 229–244). Washington, DC: Armed Forces Institute of Pathology.

Emory University Winship Cancer Institute. (2003). *CancerQuest.* Retrieved November 27, 2003, from http://www.cancerquest.org

Foltz, A.T., & Mahon, S.M. (2000). Application of carcinogenesis theory to primary prevention. *Oncology Nursing Forum, 27*(Suppl. 9), 5–11.

Giarelli, E., Jacobs, L., & Jenkins, J. (2002). Cancer prevention, screening & early detection: Human genetics. In K. Jennings-Dozier & S.M. Mahon (Eds.), *Cancer prevention, detection, and control: A nursing perspective* (pp. 99–141). Pittsburgh, PA: Oncology Nursing Society.

Hanahan, D., & Weinberg, R.A. (2000). The hallmarks of cancer. *Cell, 100,* 57–70.

Harris, L.L. (2000). Head and neck malignancies. In C.H. Yarbro, M.H. Frogge, M. Goodman, & S.L. Groenwald (Eds.), *Cancer nursing: Principles and practice* (5th ed., pp. 1210–1243). Sudbury, MA: Jones and Bartlett.

Hermans, R. (Ed.). (2001). *The encyclopaedia of medical imaging: Head and neck imaging* (Volume VI 2). Retrieved December 22, 2003, from http://www.amershamhealth.com/medcyclopaedia

Hoffman, H.T., Karnell, L.H., Robinson, R.A., Pinkston, J.A., & Menck, H.R. (1999). National Cancer Data Base report on cancer of the head and neck: Acinic cell carcinoma. *Head and Neck, 21,* 297–309.

Hong, W.K., Lippman, S.M., Itri, L.M., Karp, D.D., Lee, J.S., Byers, R.M., et al. (1990). Prevention of second primary tumors with isotretinoin in squamous-cell carcinoma of the head and neck. *New England Journal of Medicine, 323,* 795–801.

Information Ventures. (1993). Cancer initiation and promotion. *Electromagnetic Field (EMF) Health Report, 1*(2). Retrieved November 27, 2003, from http://infoventures.com/emf/hrpt/v1/n2ab2.html

Introgen Therapeutics. (2004). *Introgen announces new clinical data for Advexin and submits request to Food and Drug Administration for initiation of accelerated approval biologics license application.* Retrieved February 20, 2005, from http://www.corporate-ir.net/ireye/ir_site.zhtml?ticker=ingn&script=411&layout=7&item_id=657350

Joseph, E., & Baibak, L. (2004). *Head and neck cancer: Squamous cell carcinoma.* Retrieved November 3, 2004, from http://www.emedicine.com/plastic/topic376.htm

Khuri, F., Lee, J.J., Lippman, S.M., Kim, E.S., Cooper, J.S., Benner, S.E., et al. (2003). Isotretinoin effects on head and neck cancer recurrence and second primary tumors [Abstract 359]. *Proceedings of the American Society of Clinical Oncology, 22,* 90.

Kimball, J. (2003). *Kimball's biology pages.* Retrieved November 27, 2003, from http://users.rcn.com/jkimball.ma.ultranet/BiologyPages

Lea, D.H., Calzone, K.A., Masny, A., & Parry Bush, A.M. (2002). *Genetics and cancer care: A guide for oncology nurses.* Pittsburgh, PA: Oncology Nursing Society.

Lewis, J.E., Olsen, K.D., & Weiland L.H. (1991). Acinic cell carcinoma. Clinicopathologic review. *Cancer, 67,* 172–179.

Malins, D.C., Polissar, N.L., & Gunselman, S.J. (1996). Tumor progression to the metastatic state involves structural modifications in DNA markedly different from those associated with primary tumor formation. *Proceedings of the National Academy of Sciences, 93,* 14047–14052.

Marshall, J. (2004). *The use of anti-vascular endothelial growth factor (VEGF) targeted therapy in the treatment of colorectal cancer* [CME Monograph]. Atlanta, GA: Thomson American Health Consultants.

Mellors, R.C. (1995). *Etiology of cancer: Carcinogenesis.* Retrieved June 27, 2004, from http://edcenter.med.cornell.edu/CUMC_PathNotes/Neoplasia/Neoplasia_04.html

National Cancer Institute. (1998). *NCI research programs: Cancer biology.* Retrieved November 27, 2003, from http://plan1998.cancer.gov/RSRCH2.html

National Cancer Institute. (2003a). *Lip and oral cavity cancer (PDQ®): Treatment.* Retrieved December 22, 2003, from http://www.nci.nih.gov/cancerinfo/pdq/treatment/lip-and-oral-cavity/healthprofessional/#Section_11

National Cancer Institute. (2003b). *Oropharyngeal cancer (PDQ®): Treatment.* Retrieved December 22, 2003, from http://www.nci.nih.gov/cancerinfo/pdq/treatment/oropharyngeal/healthprofessional/#Section_9

National Cancer Institute. (2003c). *Salivary gland cancer (PDQ®): Treatment.* Retrieved November 5, 2004, from http://www.nci.nih.gov/cancertopics/pdq/treatment/salivarygland/healthprofessional

National Cancer Institute. (2004). *Laryngeal cancer (PDQ®): Treatment.* Retrieved February 20, 2005, from http://www.nci.nih.gov/cancertopics/pdq/treatment/laryngeal/HealthProfessional/page1

National Institute of Dental and Craniofacial Research. (2003). *Request for grant applications.* Retrieved November 27, 2003, from http://grants.nih.gov/grants/guide/rfa-files/RFA-DE-04-003.html

Olsen, K.D., Lewis, J.E., & Suman, V.J. (1997). Spindle cell carcinoma of the larynx and hypopharynx. *Otolaryngology—Head and Neck Surgery, 116,* 47–52.

Oral and Maxillofacial Pathology List. (n.d.). *Spindle cell carcinoma.* Retrieved December 29, 2003, from http://www.dental.mu.edu/oralpath/lesions/spindlecellca/spindlecellca.htm

Ridge, J.A., Glisson, B.S., Horwitz, E.M., & Meyers, M. (2004). Head and neck tumors. In R. Pazdur, L.R. Coia, W.J. Hoskins, & L.D. Wagman (Eds.), *Cancer management: A multidisciplinary approach* (8th ed., pp. 39–85). Manhasset, NY: CMP Healthcare Media.

Saunders, W.H., & Wakely, P. (n.d.). *Atlas of head and neck pathology.* Retrieved May 16, 2005, from http://www.medicine.osu.edu/oto/atlas.html

SEER Training. (n.d.). *Head and neck cancer: Morphology and grade.* Retrieved December 29, 2003, from http://training.seer.cancer.gov/ss_module06_head_neck/unit03_sec02_mbg.html

Slaga, T.J. (1983). Overview of tumor promotion in animals. *Environmental Health Perspectives, 50,* 3–14.

Speight, P.M., & Barrett, A.W. (2002). Salivary gland tumours. *Oral Diseases, 8,* 229–240.

Stanley, R.J., Weiland, L.H., DeSanto, L.W., & Neel, H.B. (1985). Lymphoepithelioma (undifferentiated carcinoma) of the laryngohypopharynx. *Laryngoscope, 95*(9 Pt. 1), 1077–1081.

Stennert, E., Kisner, D., Jungehuelsing, M., Guntinas-Lichius, O., Schroder, U., Eckel, H.E., et al. (2003). High incidence of lymph node metastasis in major salivary gland cancer. *Archives of Otolaryngology—Head and Neck Surgery, 129,* 720–723.

Toma, S., Bonelli, L., Sartoris, A., Mira, E., Antonelli, A., Beatrice, F., et al. (2004). 13-cis retinoic acid in head and neck cancer chemoprevention: Results of a randomized trial from the Italian Head and Neck Chemoprevention Study Group. *Oncology Reports, 11,* 1297–1305.

CHAPTER 4

Prevention and Early Detection

Margaret L. Colwill, RN, BSN, CORLN, and
Helen Lazio-Stegall, RN, BSN, CORLN

Introduction

Cancer prevention and early detection, aimed at decreasing the incidence of cancer or its severity, involve three common themes. First, an understanding of risk factors allows for appropriate lifestyle choices and more effective screening of high-risk populations. Second, cancer screening provides early detection and initiation of treatment in a timely manner. Finally, ongoing research in chemoprevention aids in the development of nutritional or pharmacologic agents to prevent or suppress cancers.

Risk Factors

Silverman and Shillitoe (1998) noted that humans are exposed continually and simultaneously to a broad spectrum of biological, chemical, and physical forces. To complicate matters even more, each individual reacts somewhat differently to these forces. Heredity, age, sex, and a multitude of other modifiers condition everyone's reactions. Current evidence suggests one conclusion more strongly than any other: "there are probably multiple causes for every type of cancer" (Silverman & Shillitoe, p. 7).

Because of the location of head and neck tumors and the functions of the vital structures they invade, patients with head and neck cancer often are faced with many challenging and life-altering situations. An understanding of risk factors could lead to early detection and treatment, thereby decreasing morbidity in this patient group.

Tumors of the Upper Aerodigestive Tract

The two most prevalent risk factors for upper aerodigestive tract tumors are tobacco and alcohol use. Use of these agents accounts for 75% of oral cancers in the United States (Kucuk, 2003). The most common chemicals found in tobacco are nitrosamines, benzene, formaldehyde, polonium, and nicotine. When used, these chemicals have harmful effects on all the tissues and vital organs in which they come into contact. Cigarette smoke is composed of organic and inorganic compounds that develop as tobacco and additives are burned. "Cigarette smoke contains tar, which is made up of over 4,000 chemicals, including the 43 known to cause cancer" (American Cancer Society [ACS], 2004b). It is believed that the carcinogenic effects of tobacco initiate genetic changes and the proliferation of cell clones in the mucosa. In turn, the entire epithelial field of the upper aerodigestive tract is at increased risk for development of cancer because of these widespread genetic abnormalities.

Smokeless tobacco or snuff contains not only carcinogenic agents but also sugars, salts, and abrasives. Prolonged contact with these substances causes insult to vital structures of the oral cavity as well as gum recession, staining of teeth, and hyperkeratosis (Spence, 1991).

Smoking cigars or small, flavored cigarettes called "bidis" is increasingly popular among teenagers and young adults. Cigars typically contain between 5 and 17 grams of tobacco. Some premium brands may contain as much tobacco in one cigar as in a whole pack of cigarettes (ACS, 2004a). Because of its size, a cigar may take up to two hours to smoke, resulting in extended exposure to its carcinogenic effects.

There is also a high correlation between the use of tobacco in any form and alcohol and the development of oral cancers. Alcohol works synergistically with tobacco, increasing the assault to the upper aerodigestive tract. In addition to causing cell damage, alcohol consumption depletes the body of selenium and vitamin A and compromises the immune system, as well. These cumulative effects of alcohol use decrease the body's ability to protect itself from cancer (Virtual Hospital, 2004). A study by Blot et al. (1988) showed that subjects who smoked more than two packs of cigarettes per day and drank more than 30 alcoholic drinks per week had a 38-fold increased risk for oral cavity and oropharyngeal cancer than subjects who did not smoke or drink. Another large-scale study by Tuyns et al. (1988) reported that subjects who were heavy drinkers and smoked more than 26 cigarettes a day had a 43-fold increased risk for cancer of the larynx.

A third known risk factor for cancer of the upper aerodigestive tract is betel nut quid. Chewing betel nut quid is a popular custom in South Asia. Various ingredients, including tobacco, lime, spices, and betel nut, are placed in a betel leaf that is folded and held in the mouth for hours or sometimes days. Prolonged exposure or repeated use of this product can lead to progressive scarring in the oral cavity tissue, resulting in precancerous lesions. As a result of betel quid use, oral cavity cancers, especially of the buccal mucosa and gingiva, are the most common head and neck malignancies in India (Argiris & Eng, 2003).

Unlike other tumors of the upper aerodigestive tract, nasopharyngeal carcinomas are not clearly associated with tobacco and alcohol use but are associated with a distinct geographic distribution. Nasopharyngeal carcinomas represent 4.4% of squamous cell cancers of the upper aerodigestive tract and are rare in the United States (Argiris & Eng, 2003); however, it is a very common malignancy in Southern China and Southeast Asia. The possible causes include genetic and environmental factors, which may be viral or dietary (Argiris & Eng). Studies show a strong association between nasopharyngeal carcinomas and ingestion of salted fish and other preserved foods in Chinese populations, especially during childhood. An additional risk factor for nasopharyngeal carcinomas is exposure to the Epstein-Barr virus. Studies have suggested a potential role for serology testing to identify individuals at high risk for nasopharyngeal carcinomas (Argiris & Eng).

Premalignant Conditions

Many premalignant mucosal conditions in the oral cavity have clinical presentations and characteristics that are known to increase the risk for cancer. Leukoplakia is defined as a white patch or plaque that cannot be differentiated chemically or pathologically from any other diseases (Neville & Day, 2002). Early or thin leukoplakia appears as a slightly elevated grayish-white plaque that does not scrape off. It may be well defined or may blend gradually into the surrounding normal mucosa. As the lesion progresses, it becomes thicker and whiter, sometimes developing a leather-like appearance with surface fissures. "On the basis of the lowest reported annual malignant transformation rate of oral leukoplakia, it can be calculated that patients with oral leukoplakia carry a five-fold higher risk of developing oral cancer than controls" (Van der Waal, Schepman, Van der Meij, & Smeele, 1997, p. 292). Certain features are associated with an increased risk of malignant transformation, including gender (females), long duration of leukoplakia, presence of leukoplakia in the floor of the mouth or tongue, idiopathic leukoplakia in nonsmokers, presence of *Candida albicans*, and presence of epithelial dysplasia (Van der Waal et al.).

Erythroplakia refers to a red patch (a red macula or plaque with a soft, velvety texture) that cannot be defined clinically or pathologically as any other condition. Erythroplakia occurs most frequently in older men. The most common sites for erythroplakia are the floor of the mouth, lateral tongue, retromolar pad, and soft palate (Neville & Day, 2002). People with erythroplakia are at 15% greater risk for the development of head and neck cancer (Argiris & Eng, 2003).

Candida is a normal flora present in the oral cavity. Chronic hyperplastic candidiasis, however, represents an overgrowth of this fungus in the mouth causing changes in the epithelium, which may be a result of acute illness, use of certain antibiotics, immunosuppression, or xerostomia. Candidiasis presents as a creamy white base that can be scraped off, revealing an erythematous base (Hyde & Hopper, 1999). The tongue, buccal mucosa, hard or soft palate, and oral commissure are the areas of the oral cavity most affected (Martin, Chambers, & Lemon, 2004).

Oral lichen planus is a complex, chronic inflammatory disease. Although the etiology is unknown, it is thought to be a mucocutaneous autoimmune disorder. These oral lesions appear in different forms and usually are not thought to have malignant potential (Hyde & Hopper, 1999; Silverman & Shillitoe, 1998). A more aggressive form called erosive or atrophic lichen planus affects a small percentage of individuals. It can be seen as a superficial ulceration and often is very painful. It is questionable as to whether this form of lichen planus has malignant potential. If so, the rates of transformation are very low, likely less than 1% (Hyde & Hopper).

Sinonasal Tumors

Sinonasal tumors may develop in any of the following anatomic locations: maxillary, ethmoid, frontal, or sphenoid sinus; nasal cavity; or nasal vestibule. Research has shown that occupational exposure to various substances is responsible for 44% of the sinonasal tract malignancies. These substances include nickel, chromium, isopropyl oils, volatile hydrocarbons, and organic fibers found in the wood, shoe, and textile industries (Costantino, Murphy, & Moche, 2004). Wood dust, in particular, is associated with adenocarcinoma of the ethmoid sinus. Individuals with wood dust exposure have a 1,000 times higher occurrence of adenocarcinoma than the general population. Infectious agents may play a role in the development of these types of tumors (Costantino et al.).

Salivary Gland Tumors

Little information is available about the etiology of malignant salivary gland tumors (SGTs), and in most instances, no known risk factors can be identified. However, several factors have been found to be associated with an increased risk for these neoplasms (Smith & Zitsch, 2003). Low-dose radiotherapy and cumulative exposure to irradiation have been implicated as significant factors for benign and malignant SGTs (Smith & Zitsch). These tumors develop after an exposure latency of 20 years. In contrast, high-dose therapeutic radiation is not reported to be linked with the development of SGTs (Eisele & Kleinberg, 2004). Various references identify a connection between infection with Epstein-Barr virus and salivary gland neoplasms, but the evidence to support this is variable (Hoffman, Funk, & Endres, 1999; Smith & Zitsch). Although tobacco and alcohol are known for their role in cancer of other head and neck sites, they have not been found to be etiologic factors for SGTs. However, a higher incidence of Warthin tumor has been reported among smokers than nonsmokers (Hoffman et al.). Discussion exists suggesting the role various environmental factors may play in SGTs, but the evidence is inconclusive. These include skin absorption of hair dye and exposure to certain metals and minerals such as nickel alloy dust or silica dust (ACS, 2005b; Hoffman et al.).

Skin Carcinomas and Melanoma

Sun exposure is the number-one risk factor for skin cancers. Multiple factors influence the development of these cancers, including outdoor occupations, amount of exposure, natural versus artificial light, and the increased exposure to ultraviolet radiation caused by changes in the ozone. Of all the areas of the head and neck, the lower lip has the highest occurrence of cancer (Weber, Robb, & Garden, 2004).

Cheilitis, or keratosis, is a premalignant change often seen in the lip after prolonged sun exposure and should be monitored for malignant transformation (Silverman & Shillitoe, 1998). Although sun exposure appears to be the major risk factor for skin melanoma, other factors include genetic makeup, family history, immune system suppression, age, and a rare condition called xeroderma pigmentosum.

The presence of a dysplastic nevus, an atypical mole, increases one's risk of skin melanoma. Depending on age, family history, the number of dysplastic nevi, and other factors, the lifetime risk for skin melanoma is estimated at 6%–10% (ACS, 2004c). Individuals with particular skin types and coloring are most sensitive to the effects of ultraviolet radiation and are at increased risk for developing skin melanoma. This includes people with red or blond hair, freckles, and fair skin that burns easily and tans with difficulty. As opposed to cumulative sun exposure, which influences nonmelanoma skin cancer, skin melanoma risk is associated with intermittent intense sun exposure (Edman & Wolfe, 2000).

A family history of skin melanoma in one or more of a person's first-degree relatives also increases the risk of skin melanoma up to eight times more than if no family history existed. Family history of skin melanoma can be attributed to gene mutation, which has been found in anywhere from 10%–40% of families with a high rate of skin melanoma (ACS, 2004c).

Thyroid Carcinomas

It is widely accepted that radiation exposure is a carcinogen known to cause thyroid cancer. There is an association between thyroid cancer and contamination caused by radioactive fallout from atomic bomb explosions as well as nuclear reactor meltdown. Thyroid cancers also have been found in individuals given external beam radiation treatments as children for facial acne and scalp ringworm. The latent period between radiation exposure and the development of thyroid carcinomas varies from 5–25 years. Adults receiving external beam radiation for a malignancy in an area not too distant from the thyroid (e.g., Hodgkin disease and non-Hodgkin lymphoma of the head and neck) currently comprise the majority of radiation-induced thyroid cancers (Saheen, 2003). Other factors associated with papillary thyroid cancer are the roles of iodine, diet, and autoimmune thyroid disease, which are not fully understood at this time.

Human Papillomavirus

Fifteen to twenty percent of subjects with head and neck squamous cell carcinomas are nonsmokers and nondrinkers. These figures indicate the presence of other risk factors (Gillison et al., 2000). Human papillomavirus (HPV) is a DNA virus with oncogenic potential that has been associated with anogenital and cervical carcinomas. Some HPV subtypes result in high risk for malignant transformation, and patients who have experienced malignancies or premalignant conditions related to HPV may have an increased risk for developing head and neck cancer (Argiris & Eng, 2003). The literature indicates that approximately 35% of all head and neck cancers and 77% of tonsillar cancers specifically harbor HPV. In addition, oropharyngeal tumors are six times more likely than other head and neck cancer sites to be HPV positive (Argiris & Eng). HPV exposure is associated with sexual risk factors such as young age at first intercourse, a history of multiple sexual partners, and a history of genital warts (Gillison et al.). Currently, various research is being done on HPV as well as the complex interaction that occurs in the virus, its host cell, and environmental factors that contribute to malignancy. The information gained from these studies may be used to intervene in and prevent the persistence of HPV infection and the impact it has in the malignant conversion of those cancers in which HPV plays a significant role (Steinberg, 2004).

Diet

The role of diet in cancer prevention is the subject of emerging research. Patients with head and neck cancer have a frequent incidence of poor-fitting dentures, loss of teeth or bone, frequent oral infections, and sores resulting from poor oral hygiene. This coupled with heavy alcohol consumption and tobacco use can lead to compromised nutrition in this patient population. It is thought that diets lacking in fruits and vegetables deplete the body of antioxidants, such as vitamins C, A, and E, beta-carotene, lycopene, selenium, and zinc. Antioxidants protect cells from the damaging effects of unstable molecules known as free radicals. There is strong support for the role antioxidants play in helping to prevent the free radical cell damage associated with cancer. Considerable laboratory evidence indicates that antioxidants may slow or possibly prevent the development of cancer. However, data from large-scale, randomized clinical trials are inconsistent (National Cancer Institute, 2004). Because patients with head and neck cancer are at high risk for poor nutrition, maintaining a healthy diet and head and neck cancer prevention are important topics for continued research.

Cancer Screening

Significant controversy exists in the literature regarding cancer screening recommendations. Debate exists regarding the benefits of generalized screening for head and neck cancers in asymptomatic subjects versus subjects at high risk. Because of easier accessibility and inspection, more focus has been paid to screening of the oral cavity and oropharynx than of the larynx (Argiris & Eng, 2003). Although there may be insufficient evidence to establish that screening results in a decrease in mortality from oral cancer, ACS recommends that an oral cavity examination be included as part of a cancer-related checkup. Similar controversy exists regarding skin cancer screening. This focuses on the benefits of population-based screening versus screening subgroups that are at higher risk for melanoma (Edman & Wolfe, 2000). In light of these issues, perhaps the better route at present is to focus on the education of healthcare workers and the general public regarding risk factor awareness.

Chemoprevention

Many cancers develop as a result of exposure to carcinogens and cancer-promoting agents. This exposure creates a stepwise accumulation of cellular and genetic changes that eventually can develop into a malignant tumor. An increased understanding of the biology of this carcinogenesis as well as the high mortality rates of recurrent disease and second primary tumors have led researchers to focus on chemoprevention.

Chemoprevention is the use of natural or synthetic chemical agents to suppress, reverse, or prevent the multistep process that leads to the formation of cancer. Primary chemoprevention uses chemopreventive agents to reverse the progression of premalignant lesions. Secondary chemoprevention focuses on preventing the development of subsequent tumors in patients

who have already received cancer-directed therapy (Kim, Hong, & Khuri, 2002).

The principles of chemoprevention in epithelial carcinomas of the head and neck are built on the concepts of multistep carcinogenesis and field cancerization. Field cancerization describes the diffuse DNA damage and epithelial differentiation caused by fieldwide exposure to carcinogens. The theory suggests that the entire epithelial surface of the upper aerodigestive tract is at increased risk for the development of premalignant and, in turn, malignant lesions (Reith & Sudbo, 2002).

Second primary tumors have become the leading cause of mortality in early-stage head and neck cancer and are an excellent example of field cancerization. Second primary tumors had previously been thought to be histologically independent from the primary tumor. As more is known about the epithelial field changes often observed in patients with head and neck cancer, second primary tumors have been found to be genetically related to the primary tumor (Wirth, Haddad, & Posner, 2003). Studies of precancerous lesions of the head and neck have been a particular focus for chemoprevention research for a variety of reasons. Premalignant oral lesions (e.g., leukoplakia, erythroplakia) associated with carcinogen exposure are known to be precursors of malignant tumors and are easily accessible for observation (Papadimitrakopoulou, 2002). Although advances in multidisciplinary cancer treatment have slightly improved the mortality rate from epithelial malignancies since the mid-1970s, the development of locally recurrent disease and second primary tumors continues to affect the morbidity and mortality of this patient population. Because of the prevalence of field cancerization in head and neck cancers, local treatment in the form of surgical excision may not be effective in preventing local recurrence or second primary tumors. Systemic action using chemoprevention agents is thought to be a better approach (Reith & Sudbo, 2002).

Numerous substances such as α-tocopherol (vitamin E), selenium, interferon, antioxidants found in fruits and vegetables, zinc, and nonsteroidal anti-inflammatory drugs are being investigated as potential systemic agents that may interrupt or inhibit the development of head and neck cancers (Kucuk, 2003). Retinoids, however, have become the main focus of this chemoprevention research because of their inhibiting effect on tumor cell proliferation and their ability to normalize cell differentiation of malignant and premalignant lesions (Contreras Vidaurre, Bagan Sebastian, Gavalda, & Torres Cifuentes, 2001).

Vitamin A, or retinol, functions in the body to regulate normal growth and differentiation of a wide variety of cell types, particularly the epithelial cells of the respiratory and digestive tracts, the nervous and immune systems, skin, and bone. Animals with vitamin A deficiencies have been shown to have a higher incidence of cancer and increased susceptibility to carcinogens (Miller, 1998).

Vitamin A can be obtained in the diet from animal sources as preformed retinoids (retinyl-esters) or from plant sources such as provitamin carotenoids, including beta-carotene. These sources are converted to retinol in the intestine and stored in the liver. Naturally occurring retinol derivatives include all-transretinoic acid (tRA) (tretinoin), 13-cis-retinoic acid (13cRA) (isotretinoin), 9-cis-retinoic acid (9cRA), and retinal (vitamin A aldehyde) (Miller, 1998). Research involves the use of these various natural and synthetic derivatives alone or in combination.

The results of research to date suggest that retinoids might be effective at suppressing the formation of head and neck cancers. Primary prevention studies (designed to reverse the progression of premalignant lesions) have demonstrated regression of leukoplakia with various response rates resulting from the use of retinol, beta-carotene, or a combination of the two (Contreras Vidaurre et al., 2001; Kim et al., 2002). Secondary prevention studies using beta-carotene and other retinol derivatives also have shown decreased incidences of second primary head and neck tumors (Contreras Vidaurre et al.). Although the retinoid compounds indicated relatively good overall response rates, the most notable issues that evolved from these studies were the high relapse rates that occurred after treatment cessation as well as the serious dose-related toxicity of vitamin A. Long-term use of high doses of vitamin A was required to achieve response, and this regimen resulted in acute and chronic toxicity. The symptoms included anorexia, weight loss, fever, hepatosplenomegaly, skin and mucous membrane changes, alopecia, cheilitis, bone and joint pain, hyperostoses, thrombocytopenia, and elevated cerebral fluid pressure. These toxicities required dose reductions, drug "holidays," or treatment cessation to resolve (Miller, 1998).

Summary

In summary, great strides have been made in showing that retinoids may have a role in the chemoprevention of head and neck carcinomas. However, questions remain concerning (a) the degree to which retinoid compounds reduce the rate of primary and secondary tumors and (b) the most effective treatment regimen (e.g., dose and treatment course regulation) that balances its chemopreventive results with its toxic side effects. Another avenue for future research is the development of other less toxic and more effective chemopreventive compounds.

References

American Cancer Society. (2004a). *Cigar smoking.* Retrieved November 8, 2004, from http://www.cancer.org/docroot/PED/content/PED_10_2X_cigar_smoking.asp

American Cancer Society. (2004b, October). *Questions about smoking, tobacco, and health.* Retrieved November 8, 2004, from http://www.cancer.org/docroot/PED/content/PED_10_2x_Questions_About_Smoking_Tobacco_and_Health.asp

American Cancer Society. (2004c, May). *What are the risk factors for melanoma?* Retrieved August 25, 2004, from http://www.cancer.org/docroot/CRI/content/CRI_2_4_2X_What_are_the_risk_factors_for_melanoma_50.asp

American Cancer Society. (2005a). *Cancer facts and figures, 2005.* Atlanta, GA: Author.

American Cancer Society. (2005b). *Detailed guide: Salivary gland cancer. What are the risk factors for salivary gland cancer?* Retrieved March 19, 2005, from http://www.cancer.org/docroot/CRI/content/CRI_2_4_2X_What_are_the_risk_factors_for_salivary_gland_cancer_54.asp?rnav-cri

Argiris, A., & Eng, C. (2003). Epidemiology, staging, and screening of head and neck cancer. *Cancer Treatment and Research, 114,* 14–46.

Blot, W.J., McLaughlin, J.K., Winn, D.M., Austin, D.F., Greenberg, R.S., Preston-Martin, S., et al. (1988). Smoking and drinking in relation to oral and pharyngeal cancer. *Cancer Research, 48,* 3282–3287.

Contreras Vidaurre, E., Bagan Sebastian, J., Gavalda, C., & Torres Cifuentes, E. (2001). Retinoids: Application in premalignant lesions and oral cancer. *Medicina Oral, 6,* 114–123.

Costantino, P.D., Murphy, M.R., & Moche, J.E. (2004). Cancer of the nasal vestibule, nasal cavity, and paranasal sinus. In L.B. Harrison, R.B. Sessions, & W.K. Hong (Eds.), *Head and neck cancer: A multidisciplinary approach* (2nd ed., pp. 455–477). Philadelphia: Lippincott Williams & Wilkins.

Edman, R.L., & Wolfe, J.T. (2000). Prevention and early detection of malignant melanoma. *American Family Physician, 62,* 2277–2285.

Eisele, D.W., & Kleinberg, L.R. (2004). Management of malignant salivary gland tumors. In L.B. Harrison, R.B. Sessions, & W.K. Hong (Eds.), *Head and neck cancer: A multidisciplinary approach* (2nd ed., pp. 620–651). Philadelphia: Lippincott Williams & Wilkins.

Gillison, M.L., Koch, W.M., Capone, R.B., Spafford, M., Westra, W.H., Wu, L., et al. (2000). Evidence of a causal association between human papillomavirus and a subset of head and neck cancers. *Journal of the National Cancer Institute, 92,* 709–720.

Hoffman, H., Funk, G., & Endres, D. (1999). Evaluation and surgical treatment of tumors of the salivary glands. In S.E. Thawley, W.R. Panje, J.G. Batsakis, & R.D. Lindberg (Eds.), *Comprehensive management of head and neck tumors* (2nd ed., pp. 1147–1181). Philadelphia: W.B. Saunders.

Hyde, N., & Hopper, C. (1999). Oral cancer: The importance of early referral. *Practitioner, 243,* 753–763.

Kim, E.S., Hong, W.K., & Khuri, F.R. (2002). Chemoprevention of aerodigestive tract cancers. *Annual Review of Medicine, 53,* 223–243.

Kucuk, O. (2003). Oral preneoplasia and chemoprevention of squamous cell carcinoma of the head and neck. *Cancer Treatment and Research, 114,* 61–83.

Martin, J.W., Chambers, M.S., & Lemon, J.C. (2004). Dental oncology and maxillofacial prosthetics. In L.B. Harrison, R.B. Sessions, & W.K. Hong (Eds.), *Head and neck cancer: A multidisciplinary approach* (2nd ed., pp. 115–128). Philadelphia: Lippincott Williams & Wilkins.

Miller, W. (1998). The emerging role of retinoids and retinoic acid metabolism blocking agents in treatment of cancer. *Cancer, 83,* 1471–1482.

National Cancer Institute. (2004, July 28). *NCI fact sheet: Antioxidants and cancer prevention.* Retrieved September 14, 2004, from http://www.nci.nih.gov/newscenter/pressreleases/antioxidants

Neville, B., & Day, T.A. (2002). Oral cancer and precancerous lesions. *CA: A Cancer Journal for Clinicians, 52,* 195–215.

Papadimitrakopoulou, V.A. (2002). Chemoprevention of head and neck cancer: An update. *Current Opinion in Oncology, 14,* 318–322.

Reith, A., & Sudbo, J. (2002). Impact of genomic instability in risk assessment and chemoprevention of oral premalignancies. *International Journal of Cancer, 101,* 205–209.

Saheen, O.H. (2003). Carcinoma of the thyroid and other malignancies. In O.H. Saheen (Ed.), *Thyroid surgery* (pp. 119–145). New York: Parthenon Publishing Group.

Silverman, S., & Shillitoe, E.J. (1998). Etiology and predisposing factors. In S. Silverman (Ed.), *Oral cancer* (4th ed., pp. 9–24). London: B.C. Decker.

Smith, R.B., & Zitsch, R.P. (2003). *Salivary gland neoplasms: A clinicopathologic approach to treatment* (3rd ed.). Alexandria, VA: American Academy of Otolaryngology—Head and Neck Surgery Foundation.

Spence, W.R. (1991). *Smokeless tobacco: A chemical time bomb.* Waco, TX: Health Edco.

Steinberg, B.M. (2004). Human papillomavirus and head and neck cancer. In L.B. Harrison, R.B. Sessions, & W.K. Hong (Eds.), *Head and neck cancer: A multidisciplinary approach* (2nd ed., pp. 973–980). Philadelphia: Lippincott Williams & Wilkins.

Tuyns, A.J., Esteve, J., Raymond, L., Berrino, F., Benhamou, E., Blanchet, F., et al. (1988). Cancer of the larynx/hypopharynx, tobacco and alcohol: IARC international case-control study in Turin and Varese (Italy), Zaragoza and Navarra (Spain), Geneva (Switzerland) and Calvados (France). *International Journal of Cancer, 41,* 483–491.

Van der Waal, I., Schepman, K.P., Van der Meij, E.H., & Smeele, L.E. (1997). Oral leukoplakia: A clinicopathological review. *Oral Oncology, 33,* 291–301.

Virtual Hospital. (2004, April). *Alcohol and cancer.* Retrieved September 13, 2004, from http://www.vh.org/adult/patient/cancercenter/prevention/preventionalcohol.html

Weber, R.S., Robb, G.L., & Garden, A.S. (2004). Basal and squamous cell skin cancers of the skin of the head and neck. In L.B. Harrison, R.B. Sessions, & W.K. Hong (Eds.), *Head and neck cancer: A multidisciplinary approach* (2nd ed., pp. 560–583). Philadelphia: Lippincott Williams & Wilkins.

Wirth, L.J., Haddad, R.I., & Posner, M.R. (2003). Progress and perspectives in chemoprevention of head and neck cancer. *Expert Review of Anticancer Therapy, 3,* 339–355.

CHAPTER 5

Patient Assessment

Cindy J. Dawson, RN, BSN, CORLN

Introduction

Head and neck cancer remains a major component of cancer statistics, despite public awareness of the detrimental effects of chronic alcohol and tobacco abuse. Squamous cell carcinoma (SCC) of the head and neck is one of the most commonly occuring cancers worldwide (Spaulding, 2002). Hoffman, Hynds-Karnell, Funk, Robinson, and Menck (1998) completed a survey of the National Cancer Data Base that demonstrated from 1985–1995, head and neck cancer represented 6.6% of all cancers in the database. The National Cancer Data Base accrued its large sample of cancer cases from hospital-based cancer registries. A total of 293,022 cases of head and neck cancer were included during this period in the database.

A further element of the morbidity of these cancers is the disabling and disfiguring treatment outcomes. Curative treatment may result in loss of sensory organs, altered physiologic function when speaking, eating, swallowing, and/or breathing, and drastic alterations in physical appearance.

Most head and neck malignancies arise from the mucosal lining of the upper aerodigestive tract and the adjacent salivary glands. A patient presenting with a head and neck tumor will exhibit a variety of complaints, depending on the anatomical area involved. SCC accounts for 90%–95% of all oral cavity and oropharyngeal tumors (lip, oral cavity, pharynx, and larynx). SCC of the mucosal membranes usually appears as a whitish plaque (leukoplakia), a velvety red area (erythroplasia), or an ulcer. Adenocarcinoma is the most common histologic type found in thyroid gland malignancies (Hoffman et al., 1998). These tumors spread in area and depth and eventually invade adjacent and underlying structures. The most frequent signs and symptoms indicating head and neck cancer are shown in Figure 5-1. Care of patients with head and neck cancer is best provided by a multidisciplinary team of healthcare providers that includes head and neck surgeons, radiation oncologists, medical oncologists, radiologists, pathologists, dental prosthodontists, clinical nurse specialists, specialized nurses, speech-language pathologists, and dietitians.

Clinical Presentation

Age and gender have a significant influence on head and neck cancer statistics. The largest percentage of head and neck cancer cases occurs in people aged 60–69 (27%), with males outnumbering females 1.5 to 1 (Hoffman et al., 1998). In a survey of the National Cancer Data Base (Hoffman et al., 1998), the largest number of tumors arose in the larynx (20.8%), followed in decreasing order by the oral cavity including lip (17.6%), thyroid gland (15.8%), and oropharynx (12.3%). The major salivary glands, which include the submandibular, sublingual, and parotid glands, were the site of origin in 4.5% of cases.

Figure 5-1. Signs and Symptoms of Head and Neck Cancer*	
• Odynophagia	• Nasal obstruction
• Dysphagia	• Epistaxis
• Weight loss (unexplained)	• Facial pain
• Loose dentition; ill-fitting dentures	• Cranial neuropathies
• Oral fetor	• Secondary infections
• Trismus	• Aspiration
• Otalgia	• Fistulization
• Neck mass	• Hemorrhage
• Serous otitis media	• Airway obstruction
• Hoarseness	• Localized pain
• Ulcer fails to heal	

*Symptoms vary depending on tumor location.

Note. From "Guidelines for Patient Management" (2nd ed., p. 1370), by T.N. Teknos, J.U. Coniglio, and J.L. Netterville in B.J. Bailey (Ed.), Head and Neck Surgery—Otolaryngology, 1998, Philadelphia: Lippincott-Raven. Copyright 1998 by Lippincott-Raven. Adapted with permission.

The multiple factors involved in caring for a patient with cancer of the head and neck often require that patients complete a myriad of tasks prior to accessing care. Patients complete a comprehensive medical history questionnaire (see Figure 5-2) detailing the chief complaint for seeking care, past medical history, medications, allergies, social history, family history, and review of systems. The patient receives information regarding privacy and signs a consent to treat form. Vital signs (height, weight, temperature, pulse, blood pressure, respirations, and, when indicated, pulse oximetry) are obtained. A specific tobacco history also is obtained and is intended to trigger a conversation with the patient about smoking cessation. This survey of tobacco use includes information on whether the patient currently uses tobacco, is a former user, or has never used. The tobacco user (past or present) then defines the type, amount, and duration of use. Expression of cigarette tobacco abuse as pack-years can help to quantify the risk of medical complications.

The head and neck nurse evaluates the patient's pain using the 0–10 verbal numeric scale or the face diagram pain rating scale (Herr, Mobily, Richardson, & Spratt, 1998). A positive pain response triggers the assessment of severity, location, duration, and quality of the pain (McCaffery & Pasero, 1999). Depending on the response to the pain scale, therapeutic intervention may be required. This often is the first step in caring for a patient with cancer and aids in developing trust in the clinical team.

The nurse performs a nutritional assessment to identify and quantify potential problems, such as dysphagia, weight loss, food intolerances, and the patient's diet history. A patient who fails to meet objective criteria for nutritional health requires a dietary consultation. It is not uncommon for patients with head and neck cancer to be malnourished because of tumor interference and/or pain with swallowing, alcohol abuse, and tobacco abuse. Weight assessment should not be the only value used to define nutritional status (see Figure 5-3).

An educational assessment is performed to evaluate the patient's readiness to learn, potential barriers to learning, level of education, reading level, and preferred style of learning. Patient education begins with the initial visit and continues throughout treatment. Examples of educational assessments are available in the *Joint Commission Guide to Patient and Family Education* (Joint Commission Resources, 2003). Defining the barriers (e.g., cognitive, religious, cultural, language, communication, financial, physical, emotional), educational preferences (e.g., reading, listening, doing, observing), and readiness for the treatment regimen is imperative at the initial encounter and during subsequent visits. The patient should receive verbal and written information regarding treatment modalities at a communication level he or she is able to understand.

In addition to performing an educational assessment, the potential knowledge deficits or learning needs of the patient are identified during this session. Examples are instruction in basic health practices, issues of self-care, patient safety, infec-

tion control, the use of medical equipment, and community resources available to the patient.

There is growing concern about medical care provided to patients who are unable to make decisions for themselves. Advances in medical technology now provide a number of treatments that may prolong life. Some patients do not want these treatments, whereas others wish to take advantage of every procedure available. The nurse should inquire if the patient has an advance directive or durable power of attorney. These legal documents will help to guide healthcare providers and caretakers in further medical treatment when the patient is unable to participate in decision making. A copy of the advance directive or durable power of attorney should be placed in the patient's medical record. If these documents are not available, the physician should document any conversations with the patient identifying his or her wishes. Information on obtaining advance directives also should be made available.

Comprehensive Health History

Present Illness

The history of the present illness for head and neck cancer is similar to a general patient history. A careful and deliberate search for the onset, location, quality, severity, timing/duration, context, and positive and negative modifying factors of the patient's complaint is completed. Pertinent information regarding the signs and symptoms related to head and neck cancer is obtained. A listing of pertinent negatives as well as positives can help to gauge the tumor size and/or clinical stage of the tumor. For example, a small laryngeal cancer may cause hoarseness without aspiration, dysphagia, or cough. Using a process of active listening may aid the healthcare provider in establishing a rapport with the patient. Beckman and Frankel (1984) found that physicians beginning an initial medical history listened an average of only 18 seconds before interrupting the patient with further questions. A process of listening that repeats and verifies clinical information will enhance the accuracy of the history and will increase the patient's trust.

Past Medical History

A list is prepared of current medications, including prescription and over-the-counter drugs, vitamins, and herbal preparations, and allergies, including inhalant, drug, and latex allergies. The patient should be questioned about any past medical conditions, with emphasis on major illnesses or injuries, hospitalizations, and surgeries. Record any implants (artificial heart valves, hip prosthesis) or external devices used by the patient. Specifically ask the patient if he or she has been instructed to routinely take antibiotics prior to a procedure, such as dental work.

Figure 5-2. Medical History Questionnaire

I-2 Medical History Questionnaire
Otolaryngology-Head and Neck Surgery Department

The University of Iowa Hospitals and Clinics (UIHC) requests this information for the purpose of providing patient care. No persons outside the UIHC are provided with this information, without your consent. If you fail to provide the requested information, patient care may be impaired. Please ask for help, if you have difficulties with the questions.

● File most recent sheet of this number ON BOTTOM ●

DATE

HOSP.#

NAME

BIRTH DATE

ADDRESS

SS#

IF NOT IMPRINTED, PLEASE PRINT DATE, HOSP. #, NAME AND LOCATION

CHIEF COMPLAINT
What are you being seen for today? _____   Who is your referring doctor? _____
                                                          Please list any other physician(s) that you would like a report sent to about
How long have you had this problem? _____   your visit _____

PAST MEDICAL HISTORY
Please list all current medical problems: Please list all surgeries: Please list any other major illnesses
                                                                               and/or other injuries:
1. _____   1. _____
2. _____   2. _____   1. _____
3. _____   3. _____   2. _____
4. _____   4. _____   3. _____
5. _____   5. _____   4. _____
6. _____   6. _____   5. _____
7. _____   7. _____   6. _____
8. _____   8. _____   7. _____
9. _____   9. _____   8. _____
10. _____   10. _____   9. _____

- Do you have any implants, such as artificial heart valves or hip prosthesis? Yes _____ No _____
- Have you ever been told to take antibiotics, prior to a surgery, because of a heart condition? Yes _____ No _____

MEDICATIONS   **ALLERGIES**
Please list your current medications. Include any birth control   Do you have a latex allergy? Yes _____ No _____
pills, over-the-counter medications and/or recreational drugs: List medication and/or food allergy(ies) and reactions:

Current Medications	Dose	Frequency		Medication/Food	Reaction

SOCIAL HISTORY
What type of work do you do? _____
Do you currently drink, or have you ever drunk alcoholic beverages in the past? Yes _____ No _____
If yes, what? _____ Amount? _____ How often? _____ Last time you drank? _____
Do you now, or have you ever used tobacco, in any form? Yes _____ No _____
If yes, what? _____ Amount? _____ How often? _____ Last time you used? _____
Are you at risk for AIDS (e.g., sexual orientation, IV drug abuse, previous blood transfusion)? Yes _____ No _____
For pediatric patients:
Are all immunizations up-to-date? Yes _____ No _____
Is the child exposed to tobacco smoke in the home or daycare setting? Yes _____ No _____
Is the child in daycare? Yes _____ No _____

(Continued on reverse)
UNIVERSITY OF IOWA HOSPITALS AND CLINICS

(Continued on next page)

Figure 5-2. Medical History Questionnaire (Continued)

I-2 Medical History Questionnaire
Otolaryngology-Head and Neck Surgery Department (continued)

Pt. Name: _____

Hospital #: _____

FAMILY HISTORY
Please circle any medical problems that run in your family (grandparents, parents, siblings and/or children):

Arthritis	Asthma	Birth defects	Bleeding problems
Diabetes	Hay fever	Hearing loss	Heart disease/heart attacks
Hypertension	Immune disorder	Kidney disease	Migraines
Problems with anesthesia	Seizures	Strokes/TIAs	Thyroid disease (goiter, etc.)
Tuberculosis	Cancer – Type: _____		

Other – Explain:_____

REVIEW OF SYSTEMS – Are You Currently Having Problems With the Following (Circle Yes (Y) or No (N), as Appropriate):

Constitutional
Night sweats	Y N
Recurrent fevers	Y N
Weight loss in the past six months	Y N
Was the weight loss intentional	Y N
What is your usual weight _____ lb	

Gastrointestinal
Indigestion/pain with eating	Y N
Chronic nausea/vomiting	Y N
Liver disease (hepatitis)/jaundice	Y N
Ulcers/gastritis	Y N
Colon/stomach cancer	Y N

Psychiatric
Anxiety	Y N
Depression	Y N
Other psychiatric disorder/treatment	Y N
If yes, list:	
_____	

Eyes
Double vision	Y N
Injuries	Y N
Glaucoma	Y N
Wearing glasses/contacts	Y N

Genitourinary
Recurrent urinary tract infections	Y N
Blood in your urine	Y N
Prostate cancer (males)	Y N
Uterine/cervical cancer (females)	Y N

Endocrine
Diabetes	Y N
Thyroid disease	Y N
Hormone problems	Y N
Are you pregnant or breastfeeding	Y N

Cardiovascular
Chest pain or angina	Y N
High blood pressure	Y N
Irregular pulse	Y N
Heart murmur	Y N
Abnormal heart anatomy	Y N

Musculoskeletal
Broken Bones	Y N
If yes, list: _____	
Chronic arm/leg weakness	Y N
Arthritis	Y N

Hematologic/Lymphatic
Anemia	Y N
Hemophilia/easy bleeding	Y N
Persistent swollen glands/lymph nodes	Y N
Blood transfusions	Y N
If yes, when: _____	

Respiratory
Asthma	Y N
Chronic cough	Y N
Emphysema	Y N
Shortness of breath	Y N
Bronchitis/pneumonia	Y N
Lung cancer	Y N
Bloody sputum	Y N
Tuberculosis	Y N

Integumentary
Skin cancer	Y N
Skin disease	Y N

Neurological
Fainting spells/"blacking out"	Y N
Seizures	Y N
Difficulty with your speech	Y N
Frequent headaches/migraines	Y N
Strokes	Y N

Immunologic
Immunologic disorders/immune deficiency	Y N
Radiation treatment	Y N
If yes, please explain: _____	
_____	

_____
Signature of Patient/Person Completing This Form

_____
Date Form Completed

_____
If Person Completing This Form is Not Patient, State Relationship to Patient

Reviewing Staff Signature	Date	No Changes	Changes as Noted

UNIVERSITY OF IOWA HOSPITALS AND CLINICS

Note. Figure courtesy of Cindy J. Dawson, RN, BSN, CORLN, University of Iowa Hospitals and Clinics. Iowa City, IA. Used with permission.

Figure 5-3. Nutrition Assessment

- Purpose
  - To assess the current nutritional status of all newly diagnosed patients with head and neck cancer; to identify and provide intervention to patients in need of pretreatment nutritional enhancement; and to assess and provide intervention to patients with head and neck cancer during treatment and post-treatment.
- Procedure
  - Newly diagnosed patients with head and neck cancer
    * Assess the nutritional status of new patients with head and neck cancer on the first clinical visit. Sample questions:
      • How would you describe your diet/nutritional status?
        - Poor, probably inadequate, adequate, or excellent
      • Have you experienced a weight loss over the past two to three months?
        - If yes, was the weight loss intentional?
      • Do you have difficulty or pain when chewing and/or swallowing your food?
        - If yes, has this caused you to change the types or consistency of the food you eat?
      • What do you eat in a normal day?
    * Provide the patient with the appropriate educational materials if nutritional status warrants.
      • "Healthy Eating Plan"
      • "High Protein, High Calorie Diet"
      • "Soft Ground and Blended Diet Guidelines"
      • "Mechanically Altered Diet"
      • "Pureed Diet"
      • "Food Tips"
    * Provide the patient with information regarding available nutritional supplements. Instruct the patient to eat or drink supplement snacks between meals, two to four times per day.
    * Instruct the patient to monitor his or her weight every other day.
    * Consult a dietitian for more detailed assessment and intervention as needed.
    * Patients undergoing treatment or post-treatment:
      • Monitor weight on every clinical visit.
      • If weight loss has occurred, assess compliance with diet, noting any difficulty eating or swallowing or complications with enteral feedings.
      • Provide intervention as needed (e.g., consult dietitian, use written nutritional materials, assess need for supplements).

Note. From *Iowa Head and Neck Protocols* (p. 563), by H. Hoffman, G. Funk, T. McCulloch, S. Graham, C. Dawson, K. Fitzpatrick, et al. (Eds.), 2000, San Diego, CA: Singluar Publishing Group. Copyright 2000 by Singular Publishing. Adapted with permission.

Psychosocial/Cultural History

A psychosocial assessment includes information about the patient's lifestyle, occupation, activities of daily living, and religious beliefs. The patient's responses are recorded on the patient questionnaire (see Figure 5-2). The use of tobacco, alcohol, and other substances is reviewed. Often, patients are unwilling to provide an accurate estimate of alcohol consumption. The nurse should guide the discussion and question the patient about the frequency of use and amounts of beer, hard alcohol, or wine. Nonjudgmental questioning with the intentional use of high estimates may yield more accurate information. Determine whether the patient is at risk for AIDS (e.g., homosexual activity, IV drug abuse, previous blood transfusion). Assess the patient's occupation for any contributing role it may play in the diagnosis. The implication of the diagnosis and treatment of cancer on the patient's return to work and the effect on the family should be addressed because they often are foremost in the minds of both the patient and family. The cultural background of patients may play a role in the diagnosis and treatment of head and neck cancer. The patient's culture may influence his or her willingness to accept the diagnosis and proposed treatment.

Family Medical History

The patient's family history completes the medical picture of the patient (see Figure 5-2). Question the patient about any family members who have been diagnosed with cancer or cardiac, pulmonary, renal, or endocrine disorders.

Review of Systems

A review of systems of the body can provide valuable information regarding concomitant medical diagnoses and may raise suspicions of metastatic disease. An example of a complete listing is presented in Figure 5-4 (DeGowin, 1994).

Physical Examination

A comprehensive head and neck examination is performed by inspection, auscultation, and palpation to evaluate potential physical causes of the patient's complaints. The following are included in a complete physical examination.
- Vital signs
  - Blood pressure—sitting, standing, and lying
  - Pulse rate and regularity
  - Respiration
  - Temperature
  - Height
  - Weight
  - Pulse oximetry, when indicated
- General assessment
  - Development
  - Nutrition
  - Body habitus (physique; general description of appearance)
  - Grooming
  - Ability to communicate

Figure 5-4. Patient Review of Systems

1. Integument—Color, pigmentation, temperature, moisture, eruptions, pruritus, scaling, bruising, bleeding
   Hair—Color, texture, loss or growth, distribution
   Nails—Color, changes, brittleness, ridging, pitting, curvature
2. Lymph nodes—Enlargement, pain, suppuration, draining sinuses, location
3. Bones, joints and muscles—Fractures, dislocations, sprains, arthritis, myositis, pain, swelling, stiffness, migratory distribution, degree of disability, muscular weakness, wasting, or atrophy, night cramps
4. Hematopoietic system—Anemia (type, therapy, response), lymphadenopathy, bleeding (spontaneous, traumatic, familial)
5. Endocrine system—History of growth, body configuration and weight, size of hands, feet, and head, especially changes during adulthood. Hair distribution. Skin pigmentation. Weakness. Goiter, exophthalmos, dryness of skin and hair, intolerance to heat or cold, tremor. Polyphagia, polyuria, glycosuria. Secondary sex characteristics, impotence, sterility treatment.
6. Allergic and immunologic history—Dermatitis, urticaria, angioneurotic edema, eczema, hay fever, vasomotor rhinitis, asthma, migraine, vernal conjunctivitis. Seasonal incidence of the foregoing. Known sensitivity to pollens, foods, dust, danders, or drugs. Previous skin test results. Results of TB or other intradermal testing. Desensitization, serum injections, vaccinations, and immunizations. HIV testing or other immunodeficiency.
7. Head—Headaches, migraine, trauma, vertigo, syncope, seizures
8. Eyes—Visual loss or color blindness, diplopia, hemianopsia, trauma, inflammation, glasses, refractive surgery, or laser treatment
9. Ears—Hearing loss, tinnitus, vertigo, discharge from ears, pain, mastoiditis, ear operations
10. Nose—Coryza, rhinitis, sinusitis, rhinorrhea, obstruction, epistaxis
11. Mouth—Sores on mouth or tongue, taste disturbance, dental problems or implants, dry mouth
12. Throat—Swallowing problems, hoarseness, dyspepsia, dysphagia, lump in the throat sensations, thyroid problems. Sore throats, tonsillitis, voice changes.
13. Neck—Swelling, suppurative lesions, enlargement of lymph glands, goiter, stiffness and limitation of motion
14. Breasts—Development, lactation, trauma, lumps, pains, discharge from nipples, gynecomastia, changes in nipples
15. Respiratory system—Pain, shortness of breath, wheezing, dyspnea, nocturnal dyspnea, orthopnea, cough, sputum, hemoptysis, night sweats, pleurisy, bronchitis, tuberculosis (history of contacts), pneumonia, asthma, other respiratory ailments
16. Cardiovascular system—Palpitations, tachycardia, irregular heartbeat, pain in the chest, exertional dyspnea, orthopnea, cough, cyanosis, ascites, edema. Intermittent claudication, cold extremities, phlebitis, postural or permanent skin color changes. Hypertension, rheumatic fever, chorea, syphilis, diphtheria.
17. Gastrointestinal system—Appetite, changes in weight, dysphagia, nausea, eructations, flatulence, abdominal pain or colic, vomiting, hematemesis, jaundice (pain, fever, intensity, duration, color of urine and stools), stools (color, consistency, odor, gas, cathartics), hemorrhoids. Changes in bowel habits.
18. Genitourinary system—Color of urine, polyuria, oliguria, nocturia, dysuria, hematuria, pyuria, urinary retention, urinary frequency, incontinence, pain or colic, passage of stones or gravel. Menstrual history—Age of onset, frequency, regularity, and duration of periods. Pregnancy—Number, miscarriages, abortions, stillbirths, deliveries, complications. Venereal history.
19. Nervous system—Cranial nerves: (a) Disturbances of smell, (b) visual changes, (c) orofacial parethesias and difficulty chewing, (d) facial weakness and taste disturbances, (e) disturbances in hearing and equilibrium, (f) difficulties in swallowing, speech, and taste, (g) limitation in motion of neck. Motor system—Paralyses, atrophy, involuntary movements, convulsions, gait, incoordination. Sensory system—Pain, lightening pain, girdle pain, parethesia, hypesthesia, anesthesia. Autonomic system—Control of urination and defecation, sweating, erythema, cyanosis, pallor, reaction to heat and cold.
20. Mental status—Mood, anger, sleep disturbances, orientation, memory, disruption of cognitive abilities

Note. From *DeGowin & DeGowin's Diagnostic Examination* (6th ed., pp. 27–29), by R.L. DeGowin, 1994, New York: McGraw-Hill. Copyright 1994 by McGraw-Hill. Adapted with permission.

- Head and face
  - Inspect the head and face. Note scars, lesions, masses, skin texture, and color.
  - Survey the facial skeleton. Note symmetry, crepitus, step-offs, or unusual features or proportions.
  - Palpate face and note tenderness over the sinuses.
  - Examine the salivary glands. Note the amount and consistency of saliva.
  - Assess the facial nerve. Note facial symmetry and strength.
  - Eyes
    * Observe extraocular movement, evidence of nystagmus, and primary gaze alignment.
    * Note the pupil size and reactivity to light.
- Ears
  * Inspect the skin of the external ear for lesions, scars, and masses.
  * Inspect the external auditory canals and tympanic membranes using an otoscope. Note any drainage.
  * Evaluate the mobility of the tympanic membrane using a pneumatic otoscope.
  * Assess hearing with tuning forks, whispered voice, finger-rub thresholds.
- Nose
  * Inspect the external nose for lesions, masses, and scars.
  * Examine the nasal mucosa, septum, and turbinates for inflammation, mucus, pus, polyps, and obstruction.

- Oral cavity, larynx, nasopharynx
  * Inspect the lips, teeth, and gingiva.
  * Examine the oral mucosa, hard and soft palate, tongue, floor of mouth, retromolar trigone, and tonsillar pillars looking for asymmetry and lesions.
  * Evaluate the hydration of the mucosal surfaces.
  * Palpate the oral cavity for masses.
  * Examine the pharyngeal walls and pyriform sinuses for pooling of saliva, asymmetry, and lesions.
  * Perform an indirect mirror examination of the larynx, giving special attention to the mucosa, mobility, and symmetry of the true vocal folds and appearance of the false cords and epiglottis.
  * Perform a mirror examination of the nasopharynx, noting the appearance of the mucosa, adenoids, posterior choanae, and opening of the eustachian tubes.
- Neck
  - Examine the neck for overall appearance and symmetry.
  - Palpate the neck for masses, tracheal position, and crepitus.
  - Palpate the lymph nodes, noting seven levels of the nodes bilaterally (see Figure 5-5).
  - Palpate the thyroid, noting enlargement, tenderness, and masses.
- Neurologic examination
  - Test cranial nerves and note any deficits.
  - Perform a brief mental status assessment, especially noting orientation to time, person, and place and the patient's mood and affect.
  - Perform a gross assessment of hearing and balance. Ask patient if he or she can hear a normal voice and walk without difficulty.
- Respiratory system evaluation
  - Inspect the chest, noting symmetry, expansion, and respiratory effort.
  - Auscultate the lungs, especially noting breath sounds, adventitious sounds, and rubs.
- Cardiovascular
  - Auscultate the heart with special attention to abnormal sounds and murmurs.

If a suspicious lesion is found during the examination, document the appearance, location, character (ulcerated, encapsulated, smooth), size, and extent of the growth. The size of the tumor, extension to adjacent structures, evidence of spread into the cervical lymphatics, and clinical evidence of distant metastasis form the basis for the clinical staging of the tumor.

A comprehensive physical examination of a patient with potential cancer of the head and neck may require the use of flexible fiberoptic endoscopes for a more detailed examination of the nasopharynx, hypopharynx, larynx, sinuses, and esophagus. Flexible endoscopy will provide additional assess-

ment data about tumor extent and involvement of adjacent structures.

Photographic documentation of the physical findings is an important documentation tool used during the pretreatment physical examination. Photographs of superficial intraoral or pharyngeal lesions are easily obtained. Nasopharyngeal, hypopharyngeal, and laryngeal photographs are obtained during laryngoscopy. Lesions of the esophagus or hypopharyngeal lesions at the esophageal introitus may be better defined using transnasal esophagoscopy.

After completing the history and physical examination, a preliminary differential diagnosis can be made. A presentation of the findings can be made to a tumor board, as needed, but may be delayed until after a histologic diagnosis.

Diagnostic Evaluation—Histologic Diagnosis

Biopsy

In some situations, a biopsy of suspicious lesions can be performed in the office or clinic. A computed tomography (CT) scan, magnetic resonance imaging (MRI), or other ra-

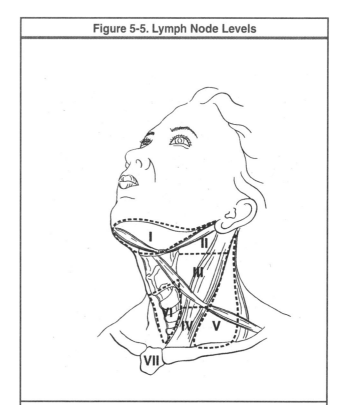

Figure 5-5. Lymph Node Levels

Note. From *AJCC Cancer Staging Manual* (6th ed., p. 19), by F.L. Greene, D.L. Page, I.D. Fleming, A.G. Fritz, C.M. Balch, D.G. Haller, et al., 2002, New York: Springer-Verlag. Copyright 2002 by the American Joint Committee on Cancer. Reprinted with permission.

diographic procedure may be performed to define the lesion and surrounding anatomy without the potential distortion produced by the biopsy.

A fine needle aspiration biopsy (FNAB) of masses in the head and neck can be useful in making a diagnosis. FNAB provides cells for histologic evaluation of salivary gland neoplasms and enlarged lymph nodes. The pathologist may be able to differentiate inflammatory, reactive, benign, and neoplastic processes with FNAB. FNAB uses a fine needle (22–25 gauge), does not seed tumor cells, and may provide a quick diagnosis.

An open biopsy of a neck mass may be done when FNAB proves to be nondiagnostic. It remains good practice to avoid an open biopsy of a neck mass as an initial step in evaluation because of the concern that the open biopsy could spread tumor cells into the neck. It is not clear whether an open biopsy of a malignant neck mass compromises survival as long as timely and appropriate treatment is initiated (Hoffman et al., 2000).

Panendoscopy

Panendoscopy of the upper aerodigestive tract is required to obtain tissue for diagnosis, screen for multiple lesions, and stage the disease. Panendoscopy usually is performed under general anesthesia in an outpatient setting. The procedures included in a panendoscopy are
- Nasopharyngoscopy
- Rhinoscopy
- Direct laryngoscopy
- Esophagoscopy
- Bronchoscopy
- Inspection and bimanual palpation of the oral cavity and neck
- Deep palpation of the base of the tongue.

Directed biopsies are done at the sites most likely to harbor a neoplasm to map the extent of any suspicious lesion (Hoffman et al., 2000). Following the endoscopic procedures and biopsies, patients are instructed to notify the physician of shortness of breath, chest pain, or hemoptysis, which may indicate a complication (see Figure 5-6).

Imaging and Other Studies

Chest x-ray is obtained to evaluate cardiopulmonary status and to review for second primary or metastatic lung tumors.

CT scan with contrast is used to evaluate the extent of disease at the primary site and to evaluate regional node status and assess adjacent bony structures.

MRI is used to evaluate tumor and lymph node status, especially in patients with poor renal function or allergy to the contrast medium. MRI is most useful in defining tumor and soft tissue relationships but does not define bony involvement well because of the low density of protons in bone.

Positron emission tomography scans are used to assess the extent of the primary lesion and the existence of recurrence or metastasis after initial therapy.

Ultrasound may be helpful for evaluating selected neck masses, especially a tumor adjacent to a vascular structure, such as the carotid artery, or a thyroid mass. The sound wave image produced by an ultrasound does not provide the level of anatomic detail visualized by other radiographic studies. It provides little information about the evaluation of a tumor's relationship to bone and cartilaginous structures. Ultrasound is not as comprehensive or definitive as CT or MRI.

Laboratory Studies
Complete blood count with differential—assesses hemoglobin and hematocrit levels, white blood cell count, especially neutrophil and lymphocyte counts, and platelets.

Electrolytes and liver function tests—detect changes in liver enzymes, electrolytes, and renal function; useful in monitoring drug toxicities.

Thyroid function tests—thyroid-stimulating hormone, T4 assesses the status of thyroid function prior to treatment of a thyroid tumor. Many types of cancer treatment can affect the function of the thyroid gland; therefore, a baseline status is important.

Glucose—screens for diabetes.

Blood urea nitrogen/creatinine—assesses renal function prior to IV contrast.

Coagulation studies—assess bleeding tendency prior to therapy.

Prostate-specific antigen test—may be performed on a male with an unknown primary adenocarcinoma that is metastatic to the neck.

Urinalysis—detects proteinuria, pyuria, or urinary tract infection.

Electrocardiogram—performed in males older than 45 or females older than 50 with a history of heart problems.

Pulmonary function testing—performed on patients at risk for perioperative complications or potential lung disease.

Diagnostic Evaluation—Consultations

Concomitant medical diagnoses are addressed as part of the complete diagnostic evaluation. Consultations that may be required include the following.
- Internal medicine—assists in the management of general medical problems (e.g., chronic obstructive pulmonary disease, hypertension, diabetes mellitus) prior to, during, and after the cancer treatment.
- Anesthesia—evaluates the patient for prolonged and extensive anesthesia that is needed during ablative and reconstructive surgery.
- Radiation oncology—evaluates the role of radiotherapy in the cancer treatment.

Figure 5-6. Homecare Instructions—Panendoscopy

B-19b₁ **HOME CARE INSTRUCTIONS**
FOR PATIENTS

DEPARTMENT OF NURSING

• File most recent sheet of this number CN BOTTOM •

DATE
HOSP. #
NAME
BIRTH DATE
ADDRESS
SS#

IF NOT IMPRINTED, PLEASE PRINT DATE, HOSP. #, NAME AND LOCATION

INSTRUCTIONS:

ESOPHAGOSCOPY/PANENDOSCOPY

Take your temperature every four hours, while awake for the next 48 hours.

Warning Signs:

If you have any of these warning signs, **do not eat or drink** and contact your doctor immediately:

—Early signs of respiratory distress: increased respiratory rate, labored breathing, or shortness of breath.
—Spitting up bright red blood.
—Fever greater than 101°F or 38.3°C.
—Chest pain.

Your throat may be sore and it may hurt to swallow for several days. A mild pain medication may be taken as prescribed by the doctor to relieve pain. If pain is not relieved, contact the doctor.

To decrease discomfort with swallowing, it may be helpful to take pain medication about ½ hour prior to meals. Call the doctor if unable to eat or drink. You should drink 1-2 quarts of liquids daily to meet your fluid needs.

Do not take aspirin or aspirin-containing medication as aspirin increases the incidence of bleeding.

Humidification with a room humidifier is helpful to reduce dryness in the mouth and throat.

Sleeping with your head elevated may be more comfortable.

Resume normal activity and/or return to work as long as vigorous activity is avoided for 48 hours.

PRESCRIPTIONS: filled _____ sent _____

DIET:

Liquids and soft foods advance to regular foods as tolerated.

SUPPLIES:

Thermometer

IF THE FOLLOWING OCCURS:
See Warning Signs

CONTACT: Call your local physician, OR

Monday-Friday (8:00 a.m.-5:00 p.m.) call ....
.... clinic at ....
OR
Weekends, nights and holidays call the hospital operator at 319/356-1616, and ask the operator
to page ....
Dr. .... is your staff doctor.

RETURN APPOINTMENT: _____

Sent with patient _____ To be notified _____

OTHER: _____

B-19b

C LABORATORY

D X-RAY EXAM

E CONSULTATION

F SPEC. EXAM

G THERAPY

H PATHOLOGY

I

PT. QUES.

SIGNATURE OF PERSON RECEIVING INSTRUCTIONS:
(I have received and understand the above instructions.)

_____
Revised: 1/01 panendo   DATE

33598/8-02

INSTRUCTIONS GIVEN BY:

_____
DATE

UNIVERSITY OF IOWA HOSPITALS AND CLINICS

WHITE—MEDICAL RECORD
YELLOW—PATIENT

Note. Figure courtesy of Cindy J. Dawson, RN, BSN, CORLN, University of Iowa Hospitals and Clinics, Iowa City, IA. Used with permission.

- Medical oncology—determines the role of chemotherapy in the overall treatment plan.
- Nutrition services—assess the patient's nutritional status and make recommendations of ways to optimize the patient before, during, and after cancer treatment.
- Social services—provide supportive services to patients and families; offer suggestions for assistance with financial, travel, and housing needs; counsel patients regarding adjustment to illness; and assist nurses and physicians with discharge planning.
- Audiology services—evaluate the patient's hearing pretreatment, especially if ototoxic chemotherapy is planned.
- Speech pathology—provides counseling and instruction for postoperative speech and swallowing problems.
- Dental/prosthodontics—evaluates and treats dental problems; counsels the patient regarding essential oral hygiene that will be required before, during, and after radiation therapy; and collaborates with the surgeon to develop prosthetic devices for reconstruction of defects.

Other referrals and evaluations that may be useful depending on the surgical procedure include

- Ophthalmology—assessment of eye/vision function with sinus tumors, for tumors in adjacent structures, or when radiation may affect orbits.
- Neurology/neurosurgery—evaluation with tumors adjacent to skull base.
- Vascular surgery—assessment if suspicion of direct vascular involvement of the tumor or necessary reconstruction following surgical resection.
- Oral surgery—evaluation for dental extraction/therapy prior to radiation.

Tumor Staging

Tumor-Node-Metastasis Classification

Accurate staging of cancer is important in determining treatment and prognosis. The tumor-node-mestasis (TNM) classification system developed by the American Joint Committee on Cancer (AJCC) (Greene et al., 2002) is based on the premise that cancers of the same anatomic site and histologic type share similar patterns of growth and outcomes (Greene et al.). The stage of the cancer correlates with the extent of the disease and prognosis for the patient.

- **T** defines the extent of the primary tumor.
- **N** is the absence or presence and extent of regional lymph node metastasis.
- **M** is the presence or absence of distant metastasis.

The use of numerical subsets of the TNM components indicates the progressive enlargement or worsening of the malignant disease.

- **Primary tumor**
  TX— Primary tumor cannot be assessed.

T0—No evidence of primary tumor
Tis—Carcinoma in situ
T1, T2, T3, T4—Increasing size of the primary tumor
- **Regional lymph nodes**
  NX—Regional lymph nodes cannot be assessed.
  N0—No regional lymph node metastasis
  N1, N2, N3—Increasing involvement of regional lymph nodes: unilateral, ipsilateral, and bilateral
- **Distant metastasis**
  MX—Distant metastasis cannot be assessed.
  M0—No evidence of distant metastasis
  M1—Distant metastasis

Further subsets of classification (e.g., T1N2bM0) are defined based on site-specific characteristics of the tumor and its biologic aggressiveness in the neck (Greene et al., 2002).

General Rules of the Tumor-Node-Metastasis Staging System

The TNM classification system is a shorthand method for describing the presentation of the malignant tumor. The following rules apply.

1. All patients should be followed through the initial course of surgery or for four months, whichever is longer.
2. All tumors must be confirmed microscopically.
3. Four classifications are described (Greene et al., 2002).
   - Clinical classification, designated as cTNM or TNM
   - Pathologic classification, designated as pTNM
   - Retreatment classification, designated as rTNM
   - Autopsy classification, designated as aTNM

Clinical Classification

Clinical assessment uses the information available before the first definitive treatment, including, but not limited to, the physical examination, imaging, endoscopy, biopsy, and surgical exploration. Clinical stage is assigned prior to any cancer-related treatment and is not changed on the basis of subsequent information. Based on AJCC guidelines, the clinical stage is essential for selecting and evaluating primary therapy for head and neck cancer (Greene et al., 2002).

Pathologic Classification

Pathologic staging uses the evidence acquired prior to treatment and is supplemented or modified by the evidence acquired from surgery, particularly the pathologic examination. The pathologic stage provides additional precise data used for estimating the prognosis of the patient and calculating end results.

Reasonable efforts to reconstruct the tumor size (pT) may be required if there have been previous biopsies or partial excision of the cancer prior to definitive surgery. The complete assessment of the regional lymph nodes (pN) ideally involves the removal of a sufficient number of lymph nodes to evaluate the highest pN status. Pathologic staging is essential to define the extent of the primary tumor and the status of regional lymph nodes. Pathologic staging depends on the proven anatomic extent of disease and whether or not the primary lesion has been completely removed.

Retreatment Classification

This new classification is made when further treatment, such as chemotherapy, is planned for a cancer that recurs following a disease-free interval. All information available at the time of retreatment should be used in determining the stage of the recurrent cancer, rTNM. Biopsy confirmation of the recurrence is useful, but with pathologic proof of the primary site, clinical evidence of distant metastasis may be used.

Autopsy Classification

This classification occurs during postmortem examination of the patient when cancer was not evident prior to death.

Stage Grouping

The TNM staging, c or p, is used to assign a patient to a specific clinical stage of disease. The larger and more disseminated the tumor, the higher the stage group and the worse the prognosis. The AJCC manual provides information that can be used to assign the clinical stage of a cancer based on the anatomic site and TNM classification. The level of TNM classification associated with a clinical stage varies for different anatomic sites. The grouping of similar TNM-classified patients ensures that each stage group is relatively homogenous for purposes of tabulation and analysis of cancer statistics and is used to discuss survival rates of the various stages.

Histopathologic Type of Cancer

The World Health Organization's "International Histological Classification of Tumours" is used to type the cancer (Fritz et al., 2000). The histologic tumor type is a qualitative assessment whereby a tumor is categorized according to the normal tissue type or cell type it most closely resembles (e.g., hepatocellular, SCC). A list of international classification of disease codes is presented in anatomic site-specific editions from the World Health Organization and can be found in the *AJCC Cancer Staging Manual* (Green et al., 2002).

Histologic Grade

The histologic grade of a cancer is a qualitative assessment of the differentiation of the tumor expressed as the extent to which a cancer resembles the normal tissue at that site (Greene

et al., 2002). The term *grade* also is used when other prognostic measures of the tissue are used for prediction, particularly nuclear grade and mitotic count.
- GX—grade cannot be assessed.
- G1—well differentiated
- G2—moderately differentiated
- G3—poorly differentiated
- G4—undifferentiated

Summary: Cancer Staging Systems

The clinical assessment of a patient with cancer can best predict outcomes of therapy when the following information has been determined:
- Anatomy—primary site
- Regional lymph node status
- Metastatic sites, if present
- Clinical and pathologic TNM classification
- Application of site-specific parameters for staging
- Stage grouping
- Histopathologic type
- Histologic grade

The clinical cancer staging assessment is an important part of the patient's medical record indicating the anatomic extent of disease. It complements a thorough history and physical examination and provides the basis to record subsequent treatment and follow-up (see Figure 5-7).

Some tumors are more accessible to clinical evaluation and can be measured, but in areas not as accessible, such as the larynx, the tumor diameter may be more difficult to measure and less significant than the extension of the tumor to adjacent sites or its impact on mobility.

Treatment

Tumor Board

After completion of the primary evaluation, all new patients are presented at a tumor board conference. As outlined in the

---

Figure 5-7. Head and Neck Tumor Sites

Oral cavity—mucosal lip, buccal lip, lower alveolar ridge, upper alveolar ridge, retromolar gingiva (retromolar trigone), floor of the mouth, hard palate, anterior two-thirds of the tongue (oral tongue)

Pharynx—nasopharynx, hypopharynx, and oropharynx (posterior one-third of tongue, tonsil, base of tongue)

Larynx—supraglottis, glottis, and subglottis

Nasal cavity and paranasal sinuses

Major salivary glands—parotid, submandibular, and sublingual

Thyroid gland

Iowa Head and Neck Protocols (Hoffman et al., 2000), the goals of a tumor board are to

1. Gather all pertinent diagnostic material regarding individual cases to permit review.
2. Assign a recommended treatment plan and offer reasonable alternatives.
3. Assign definitive staging.
4. Create an interactive environment to foster communication between specialties.
5. Teach the participating staff, fellows, and resident physicians.
6. Teach medical students.
7. Provide a forum in which second opinions are routinely offered.
8. Develop or add to a detailed cancer database.

The attendees include all specialized team members who have evaluated the patient. Core members of the tumor board for all cases presented are head and neck surgeons, radiation oncologists, diagnostic radiologists, pathologists, dental prosthodontists, medical oncologists, oncology nurses, oncology social workers, and speech-language pathologists. The team provides input regarding the best treatment plan for the patient. A TNM staging form is completed for the primary site of the tumor with the pathology defined for T, N, M, and stage. A consensus for treatment is gathered from all tumor board members for presentation to the patient and family. Treatment options may include surgery, radiation, chemotherapy, or a combination of any of the three. The consequences of no further treatment also are discussed.

Patient and Family Counseling

The head and neck surgeon presents the results of the diagnostic evaluation and tumor board recommendations to the patient and family in a compassionate but direct fashion. An inclusive review of the patient's options is presented with emphasis on a balanced and complete picture of all treatment modalities—surgery, radiation therapy, chemotherapy, or combined modalities of treatment. A thorough and impartial appraisal of the patient's treatment options and alternatives is essential to reduce any "framing bias" about the risks and benefits of therapy for this cancer (Gordon-Lubitz, 2003). Risk perception is affected not only by patient factors (e.g., sex, prior beliefs, past experience) but also by how the treatment information is presented. A combination of visual displays, statistical information with individualized risk estimates, and qualitative explanations of therapy is necessary to obtain informed consent.

A description of the result of surgical therapy often is followed by the benefits of reconstructive techniques. Informed consent should be regarded as a crucial educational, interactive tool that encourages patients to accept certain responsibilities (Saxton, 2003). When properly applied, an informed consent can place the patient's expectations at a more manageable and realistic level. It also can reduce the risk of liability of potentially disfiguring surgery by educating the patient and family about the complications that can occur and the importance of deciding whether the offered procedure is worth the risk. Should the patient decide on no further treatment, a thorough discussion about the natural progression of the cancer also is necessary. The intensity level of this discussion warrants the involvement of family or significant others. Often, it is desirable to schedule a follow-up appointment to repeat the information and answer subsequent questions once the patient and family have had time to evaluate the options. The need to offer a second opinion should be balanced against the nature or extent of the cancer and the desire for the timely treatment of the cancer. If the tumor is advanced, a delay in treatment to obtain a second opinion may compromise patient survival. So much information is provided at this time that it often is hard for both the patient and physician to remain focused. A simple checklist in the patient chart can document that the patient received the necessary information during the assessment (see Figure 5-8). Many physicians have a nurse witness the informed consent procedure. It is the nurse's role to review the informed consent process and operative consent form and to ask the patient and family three questions.

- Have you read this form or has it been read to you?
- Do you understand the information provided on this form?
- Do you have any further questions?

By reviewing this form, the nurse witness specifically verifies that the patient has read the form, understood it, and had all of his or her questions answered.

The head and neck oncology nurse specialist coordinates and facilitates patient care among multiple disciplines within the healthcare facility and the local community, including home health agencies, referring physician, and other community support services. As an educator, the nurse initially provides information to the patient and family on the cancer diagnosis, reducing risk factors, diagnostic tests and procedures, recommended therapy, consequences, and side effects. During treatment and follow-up, education focuses on changes to body image, nutrition, functional support, quality of life, and symptom management. A major nursing role is coordinating and attending weekly tumor board conferences. In coordinating the head and neck tumor board, the nurse specialist reviews the patient list, confirms attendance with pertinent specialties, compiles cancer staging decisions, arranges pretreatment consultation, and serves as a resource for the patient and family. Another role is attending multidisciplinary rounds on the inpatient unit along with speech pathology and dietary. The rounds address patient progress, discharge planning issues, and follow-up needs. Discussion of future surgical patients also is presented. The nurse also is an integral participant in research activities in head and neck oncology. The head and neck nurse specialist helps to iden-

Figure 5-8. Sample Check-Off Sheet			
Check-Off Sheet **Documents the written/verbal teaching and diagnosis materials provided and recommendations**	**Document**	**Date**	**Initials**
	Summary of tumor board		
	Clinical indicators reviewed		
	Teaching material provided		
	Illustration of surgery		
	Smoking cessation/substance abuse information		
Complete these documents as the patient proceeds through cancer workup and treatment.	Surgical plan reviewed		
	Post-op care instructions		
	Informed consent		
	Witness		
	Second opinion		

tify potential patient participants for studies and implements protocol into the patient's treatment plan.

Treatment Modalities

In an analysis of head and neck cancer between 1985 and 1994 (Hoffman et al., 1998), surgery was the most common treatment for cancers of the lip, thyroid gland, and oral cavity. Radiation was the most common treatment for cancers of the nasopharynx, larynx, and oropharynx. Combined surgery and radiation therapy was the most common treatment for cancers of the major salivary glands and hypopharynx. Combined chemotherapy and radiation therapy was used to treat nasopharyngeal, hypopharyngeal, and oropharyngeal cancers.

Treatment considerations are based on tumor factors, such as anatomical site, size, extent or stage of cancer, and the tumor type. Patient factors, such as medical status, age, occupation, comorbidities, previous therapy, patient's wishes, social habits, and reliability for follow-up, also are considered when determining treatment options. Treatment goals should include complete removal of the cancer, satisfactory post-treatment functioning, and an acceptable cosmetic result.

Summary

The clinical presentation, diagnostic evaluation, tumor staging, and treatment recommendations for the patient with head and neck cancer is a complex and comprehensive process. A flow chart delineating the assessment pathway of the typical patient is presented in Figure 5-9. A comprehensive evaluation and treatment recommendation provides the patient and family with the best treatment options for a difficult and complicated disease.

References

Beckman, H.B., & Frankel, R.M. (1984). The effect of physician behavior on the collection of data. *Annals of Internal Medicine, 101,* 692–696.

DeGowin, R.L. (1994). *DeGowin & Degowin's diagnostic examinations* (6th ed.). New York: McGraw-Hill.

Fritz, A., Percy, C., Jack, A., Shanmugaratnam, K., Sobin, L., Parkin, D.M., et al. (Eds.). (2000). *International classification of disease for oncology* (3rd ed.). Geneva, Switzerland: World Health Organization.

Gordon-Lubitz, R.J. (2003). Risk communication: Problems of presentation and understanding. *JAMA, 289,* 95.

Greene, F.L., Page, D.L., Fleming, I.D., Fritz, A.G., Balch, C.M., Haller, D.G., et al. (Eds.). (2002). *AJCC cancer staging manual* (6th ed.). New York: Springer-Verlag.

Herr, K., Mobily, P., Richardson, G., & Spratt, K. (1998). *Use of experimental pain to compare psychometric properties and usability of pain scales in the adult and older adult populations.* Research presentation at the American Society for Pain Management in Nursing annual meeting, Orlando, Florida.

Hoffman, H., Funk, G., McCulloch, T., Graham, S., Dawson, C., Fitzpatrick, K., et al. (Eds.). (2000). *Iowa head and neck protocols.* San Diego, CA: Singular.

Hoffman, H.T., Hynds-Karnell, L., Funk, G., Robinson, R., & Menck, H. (1998). The National Cancer Data Base report on cancer of the head and neck. *Archives of Otolaryngology—Head and Neck Surgery, 124,* 951–962.

Joint Commission Resources. (2003). *Joint Commission guide to patient and family education.* Oakbrook Terrace, IL: Author.

McCaffery, M., & Pasero, C. (1999). *Pain: Clinical manual* (2nd ed.). St. Louis, MO: Mosby.

Saxton, J.W. (2003). *The satisfied patient: A guide to preventing malpractice claims by providing excellent customer service.* Marblehead, MA: HCPro Press.

Spaulding, M.B. (2002). Recent advances in the treatment of head and neck cancer. *ORL—Head and Neck Nursing, 20*(1), 9–15.

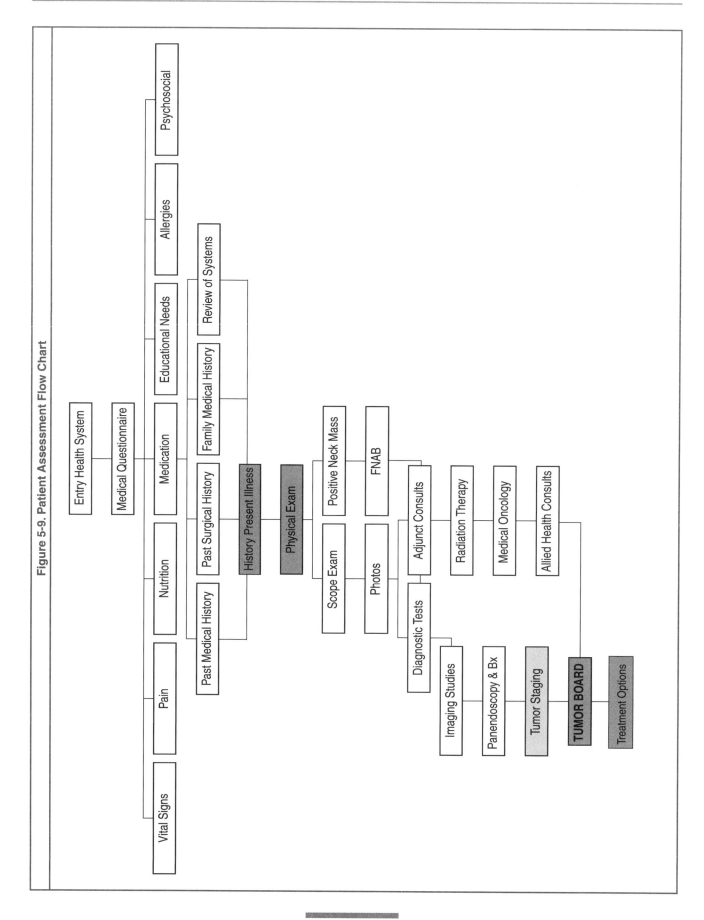

Figure 5-9. Patient Assessment Flow Chart

CHAPTER 6

Surgical Management of Head and Neck Malignancies

Raymond Scarpa, MA, CNS, AOCN®, and
Jose Zevallos, BA

Introduction

Surgery remains one of the most important treatment modalities for tumors of the head and neck. Although viewed as a cornerstone in the management of head and neck cancers, surgical intervention has limits. Its limits are defined by the extent of the tumor, the functional and cosmetic defects that can result from the surgery, and the skill and experience of the surgeon.

Treatment of tumors that are limited in size and confined to their primary site may be best managed with the use of surgery alone. The oncologic standard of surgical intervention is to remove the primary tumor with a 2-cm margin of tumor-free tissue around the primary site. Early lesions (T1 and T2 in the American Joint Committee on Cancer tumor-node-metastasis [TNM] staging system) are most amenable to conservative surgical intervention with favorable cosmetic and functional outcomes.

Treatment of patients with more locally advanced lesions (T3 and T4) and of those with lymphatic node metastases generally requires combined modalities. Radiation and chemotherapy play vital roles in determining favorable treatment outcomes when combined with appropriate and timely surgical intervention for these locally advanced lesions.

Some advanced lesions in the head and neck area may require palliative surgical management (along with combined adjuvant treatment modalities). Surgical debulking may be indicated to provide functional or symptomatic relief from lesions that invade or compress vital structures in the head and neck. Intentional surgical debulking is not commonly performed and seldom is indicated, except as a palliative resection for patients with distant metastases.

The goals of surgical management of head and neck tumors are to remove the tumor, restore function, and preserve cosmetic appearance. Radical surgical resections may result in both cosmetic and functional defects. Surgical reconstruction using various tissue flaps and grafts helps to restore these defects. The following sections will discuss surgical resection and reconstruction of selected tumors in the head and neck and will address functional and cosmetic outcomes of the various procedures.

Neck Dissection

The term *neck dissection* refers to the surgical removal of cervical lymph nodes in various levels of the neck. This generally is performed in conjunction with surgical resection of the primary tumor in the upper aerodigestive tract. This section will review the anatomic levels of the neck and corresponding groups of lymph nodes in each level. It also will review the classifications of neck dissections, surgical management, and the procedure of choice for selected primary lesions.

Indications for any of the various types of neck dissection depend on the size, location, and cell makeup of the primary site and the lymphatic drainage pattern associated with that site. Other issues include clinical evidence of disease in the neck before or after other treatment modalities are implemented and the likelihood that metastatic disease will occur or is present microscopically in a group(s) of corresponding lymph nodes at a specific level in the neck.

The status of cervical lymphadenopathy, cervical lymph node metastases, in patients with squamous cell carcinoma of the aerodigestive tract is a significant prognostic indicator. Rates for cure tend to drop by nearly half when regional lymph nodes are involved (Muller, Newlands, Quinn, & Ryan, 2002).

Lymph Node Levels and Groups

In his 1938 paper "Anatomy of the Human Lymphatic System," H. Rouvier described the routes of lymphatic drainage in the head and neck. Since that time, many systems have been developed to describe the regional lymph nodes of the head and neck area (Dubner, 2004).

The system developed by the Head and Neck Service at Memorial Sloan-Kettering Cancer Center provided a description of regional nodes that is subdivided into levels with clinical descriptions. In the monograph "Pocket Guide to Neck Dissection Classification and TNM Staging of Head and Neck Cancer" by Robbins (2001), classifications were published that reflect this system (see Figure 6-1). Figure 6-2 shows the levels of the neck.

Neck Dissection Classifications

In 1906, Dr. George Crile described the importance of surgically removing metastatic disease in the neck (Crile, 1987). His technique, known as radical neck dissection (RND), included removal of the lymph nodes from levels I–V, the submandibular gland, the internal jugular vein, and the spinal accessory and greater auricular nerves. It also included removal of the digastric, stylohyoid, and sternocleidomastoid muscles (SCM). The operation described by Crile remains the benchmark to which all modifications are compared (Dubner, 2004).

Trends toward conservative surgery began to develop in the 1960s and '70s. Surgical techniques were developed to address cosmetic and functional limitations that resulted from RND. Nomenclature describing modifications to RND created some misunderstanding, necessitating a standardized system to address modifications to the procedure.

In 1991, the Committee for Neck Dissection Classification, composed of the American Head and Neck Society and the Committee for Head and Neck Surgery and Oncology of the American Academy of Otolaryngology—Head and Neck Surgery, developed a classification system for neck dissections to address this issue, which was revised in 2002 (Robbins et al., 1991, 2002). The following terminology regarding classifications for neck dissection reflects this work.

Radical Neck Dissection

RND involves removal of the internal jugular vein, the SCM, the submandibular gland, the spinal accessory and greater auricular nerves, and all lymphatics from levels I–V. This procedure is indicated when extensive metastatic disease is present in the neck, including direct extension to any of the structures in the neck or extension of disease beyond the capsule of a lymph node.

A significant cosmetic deformity results from removal of the SCM, namely a flat deformity to the contour of the neck on the affected side. However, patients experience little to no limitation in range of motion to the neck. Sacrifice of the spinal accessory nerve leads to significant cosmetic and functional consequences. Significant limitation in range of motion to the affected shoulder occurs. Deinnervation of the trapezius muscle can lead to chronic pain, shoulder droop, muscle atrophy, and shoulder fixation (Shah & Patel, 2003).

Figure 6-1. Classifications of Lymph Node Groups by Level

Level I:
Submental—At significant risk for metastatic disease from primary tumors arising from the floor of the mouth, anterior tongue, mandibular alveolar ridge, and lower lip
Submandibular—At significant risk for metastatic disease from primary tumors arising from the oral cavity, nasal cavity, mid-face soft tissue structures, and submandibular gland
Ia: The submental triangle
Ib: The submandibular triangle

Level II:
Upper jugular area—Primary cancers arising from the nasopharynx, hypopharynx, oropharynx, larynx, oral cavity, nasal cavity, and parotid gland pose the greatest risk for metastatic disease in this level.
IIa: Found in the upper one-half of the superior jugular area. The lower border is the spinal accessory nerve.
IIb: Found in the lower one-half of the upper jugular area

Level III:
Middle jugular area—Primary cancers arising from the nasopharynx, hypopharynx, oropharynx, larynx, and oral cavity pose the greatest risk for metastatic disease in this level.

Level IV:
Lower jugular area—Primary cancers arising from the hypopharynx, upper esophagus, and larynx pose the greatest risk for metastatic disease in this level.

Level V:
Posterior triangle—Primary cancers arising from the nasopharynx and oropharynx are at risk for developing metastatic disease in this level. The inferior belly of the omohyoid muscle divides the subzones of Va and Vb.
Va: Includes lymphatic structures that follow the spinal accessory nerve
Vb: Includes lymphatic structures that lie along the transverse cervical artery

Level VI:
Known as the anterior compartment of the neck. It includes prelaryngeal, pretracheal, paratracheal, and precricoid lymphatic structures. Primary cancers arising from the thyroid gland, cervical esophagus, glottic and subglottic areas of the larynx, and pyriform sinus are at greatest risk for metastatic disease at this level. Nodes in this area also are known as Delphian nodes.

Note. Based on information from Robbins, 2001.

The surgical approach is made with an incision at the level of the mastoid process that extends two fingerbreadths below the angle of the mandible to the anterior part of the mandible. A second incision is made at the midpoint of the first incision over the posterior aspect of the SCM in a lazy "S" fashion down to the midclavicle. The standard neck dissection removes the fascia and lymphatics deep to the platysma *en bloc* from levels I–V. It also removes all the

Figure 6-2. Levels of the Neck

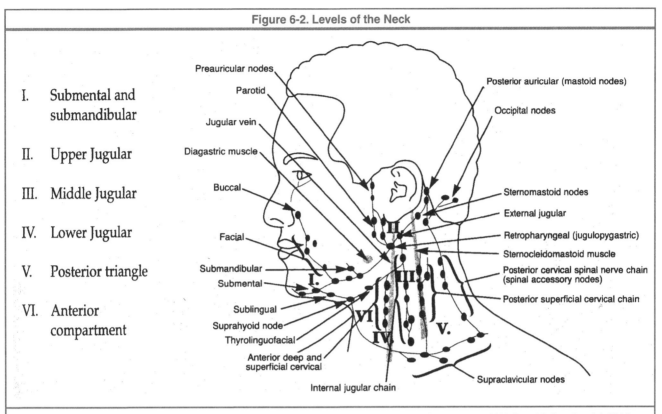

I. Submental and submandibular

II. Upper Jugular

III. Middle Jugular

IV. Lower Jugular

V. Posterior triangle

VI. Anterior compartment

Note. From "General History, Risk Factors and Normal Physical Assessment" (p. 21), by H.G. Andresen, M.H. Cyr, J.P. Guadagnini, M.M. Hickey, T.S. Higgins, M.B. Huntoon, et al. in L.L. Harris and M.B. Huntoon (Eds.), *Core Curriculum for Otorhinolaryngology and Head-Neck Nursing,* 1998, New Smyrna Beach, FL: Society of Otorhinolaryngology and Head-Neck Nurses, Inc. Copyright 1998 by Society of Otorhinolaryngology and Head-Neck Nurses, Inc. Reprinted with permission.

nonlymphatic structures mentioned earlier (Shah & Patel, 2003) (see Figure 6-3).

Modified Radical Neck Dissection

Modified radical neck dissection (MRND) includes removal of all lymph nodes normally removed in RND with preservation of one or more of the nonlymphatic structures. This procedure is indicated in cases of extensive metastatic disease that does not involve or is not adherent to any nonlymphatic structures in the neck (Muller et al., 2002).

MRND is designed to reduce the cosmetic and functional limitations associated with RND without compromising the oncologic treatment. Sacrifice of the spinal accessory nerve in RND leads to shoulder dysfunction and neck pain. Function and pain are accentuated when postoperative radiation therapy is given. Removal of the SCM is not functionally debilitating but causes a cosmetic deformity. Sacrifice of the internal jugular vein results in facial edema because of diminished venous blood flow and compromised lymphatic drainage. Postoperative radiation therapy can lead to fibrosis of remaining tissue and lymphatic and venous systems in the area of treatment, adding to the development of facial edema.

Preservation of the internal jugular vein is an important consideration if a bilateral neck dissection is planned. If the vein must be sacrificed bilaterally, the surgeries should be staged at least one week apart to allow collateral circulation to develop (Dubner, 2004).

Extended Radical Neck Dissection

Extended radical neck dissection (ERND) involves removal of all structures included in RND with the removal of additional lymphatic and nonlymphatic structures, including the carotid artery, skin, vagus or hypoglossal nerves, and additional lymph node groups, such as the mediastinal, parapharyngeal, or paratracheal lymph nodes (Shah & Patel, 2003). ERND can leave the patient with significant functional and cosmetic impairments. The degree of impairment will vary depending on the structures removed.

Selective Neck Dissection

The term *selective neck dissection* (SND) is used when one or more lymph node groups are preserved. The basis for selective removal or preservation of various lymphatic groups depends on the primary tumor site and the predicted pattern of lymphatic spread (Robbins, 2001).

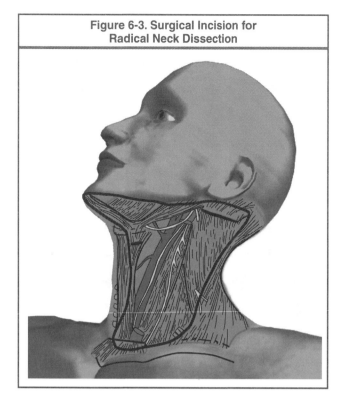

Figure 6-3. Surgical Incision for
Radical Neck Dissection

SND is classified into four types of procedures: supraomohyoid neck dissection (SOHND), lateral neck dissection, anterior neck dissection, and posterolateral neck dissection. The type of SND is determined by the specific site and initial staging of the tumor and by the general absence of palpable cervical lymph nodes.

Supraomohyoid neck dissection. SOHND is indicated for primary tumors that originate in the oral cavity between the vermilion border of the lips and the hard and soft palate junction superiorly and the circumvallate papillae of the tongue inferiorly. SOHND also can be done for tumors of the upper and lower alveolar ridges, floor of the mouth (FOM), retromolar trigone, anterior two-thirds of the tongue, and buccal mucosa (Muller et al., 2002).

Tumors arising from these areas have a high incidence of occult (nonpalpable) disease in the neck. As a result, SOHND is indicated for patients who present without clinical or radiologic evidence of disease in the neck. A bilateral SOHND is performed when the tumor crosses the midline of the primary site (Muller et al., 2002) (see Figure 6-4).

The submandibular gland on the affected side and lymphatic structures in levels I, II, and III are removed during SOHND. When the oral tongue is involved, lymphatic spread to level IV may occur, necessitating removal of the lymphatic structures in level IV (Robbins, 2001). SOHND has relatively low morbidity and is less debilitating cosmetically and functionally when compared to RND.

An incision is made in an upper skin crease starting two fingerbreadths below the angle of the mandible at the posterior

border of the SCM and extends toward the hyoid bone to the anterior portion of the neck. If an oral approach is planned for removal of the primary tumor, the lymphatics in levels I, II, and III may be removed *en bloc* (Shah & Patel, 2003).

Lateral neck dissection. Lateral neck dissection is indicated for surgically treated tumors of the oropharynx, hypopharynx, and larynx in patients with or without clinically palpable nodal disease. The procedure involves removal of the upper jugular lymph nodes from level II, midjugular lymph nodes from level III, and lower jugular lymph nodes from level IV *en bloc* for tumors that originate in the hypopharynx or larynx (Robbins, 2001). Level I lymph nodes also are removed if the primary tumor originated in the oropharynx.

The oropharynx contains the tonsils, tonsillar fossa and pillars, base of the tongue, and the posterior pharyngeal walls, and tumors tend to metastasize to the lymphatics in levels II–IV. The size of a primary oropharyngeal tumor is not a factor in its ability to metastasize (Muller et al., 2002). Functional disabilities, such as difficulty with swallowing, speaking, and breathing, can occur when extensive oropharyngeal surgery is performed. Because of these functional limitations and the difficulty in accessing these tumors, they often are treated with primary radiation therapy. The field of radiation also includes the neck (Muller et al.).

The hypopharynx is an area very rich in lymphatic tissue. Tumors in this area tend to metastasize bilaterally in the neck. The hypopharynx extends superiorly from the level of the hyoid bone and to the cricoid cartilage inferiorly. It includes the pyriform sinus, posterior cricoid mucosa, and hypopharyngeal wall.

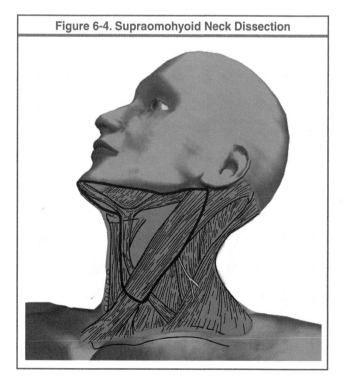

Figure 6-4. Supraomohyoid Neck Dissection

The larynx is divided into the supraglottic and glottic areas. Tumors in the supraglottis or the area above the vocal cords have the greatest potential for cervical lymph node metastasis because of a rich lymphatic supply. This potential for metastasis results in the need for surgical patients to have a bilateral SND with clinically negative neck disease. Radiation therapy is an alternative primary treatment for supraglottic tumors. Tumors of the glottis do not commonly metastasize because of sparse lymphatics and anatomic barriers, unless the tumor is large and extends to adjacent areas.

Anterior neck dissection. Anterior neck dissection involves removal of lymphatic structures from level IV and is indicated for patients with primary tumors originating in the thyroid gland, parathyroid glands, cervical esophagus, and glottic and subglottic larynx. The lymphatics in this level are known as paratracheal, Delphian, perithyroid, and pretracheal lymph nodes. The paratracheal lymph nodes are found along the right and left recurrent laryngeal nerve. The Delphian nodes are found in the precricoid area (Muller et al., 2002).

The superior limit of the dissection is the hyoid bone and the inferior limit is the suprasternal notch. The dissection is carried out laterally to the right and left carotid sheaths (Muller et al., 2002). Most patients tolerate this procedure well, with minimal cosmetic and functional disabilities, especially in combination with thyroid surgery. This procedure also is indicated for laryngeal tumors and is performed in conjunction with a laryngectomy (see Figure 6-5).

Posterolateral neck dissection. Posterolateral neck dissection is an *en bloc* procedure that removes levels II–V lymphatics and also may include lymphatics found in the suboccipital and postauricular areas. Posterolateral neck dissection is indicated primarily for patients with skin tumors. These include melanoma, squamous cell carcinoma, and soft tissue sarcoma (Muller et al., 2002).

The dissection is carried superiorly to the base of the skull, posteriorly to the nuchal ridge, inferiorly to the clavicle, medially to the lateral border of the sternohyoid and stylohyoid muscles, and laterally to the anterior border of the trapezius muscle (Robbins, 2001). Cosmetic and functional limitations are minimal if the spinal accessory nerve is preserved. The location of the primary lesion and subsequent resection may have significant cosmetic and functional deformities (see Figure 6-6).

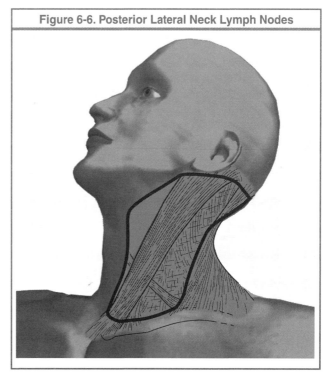

Figure 6-6. Posterior Lateral Neck Lymph Nodes

Summary: Neck Dissection

Since the original description of RND by Crile in 1906 (Crile, 1987), surgical techniques and nomenclature have been refined to include various types of neck dissection. The ability to diagnose and treat these malignancies with combined modalities, such as chemotherapy and radiation therapy, has led to improved patient outcomes. The development of positron emission tomography scanning continues to improve diagnostic abilities that will assist in directing and improving treatment plans.

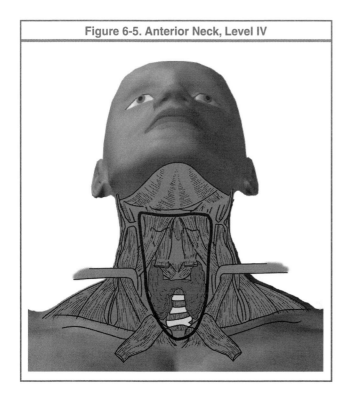

Figure 6-5. Anterior Neck, Level IV

Controversy continues to exist in the treatment of neck disease in patients with head and neck malignancies. These areas of debate include management of the carotid artery when it is involved in cervical metastases and management of the neck in patients with superficial extension of glottic tumors to the supraglottis. Other areas of debate are management of advanced disease in the neck after organ preservation therapy, management of level IV lymph nodes in the N0 neck in patients with primary lesions of the oral tongue, and sentinel node localization in squamous cell carcinomas of the head and neck (Muller et al., 2002). As research continues, classification and surgical techniques regarding neck dissection will continue to develop.

Laryngectomy

The larynx is a complex neuromuscular organ divided into three regions, the supraglottic, glottic, and subglottic areas. The supraglottic larynx starts at the superior tip of the epiglottis and extends to include the false vocal cords. This area acts as a passageway for air and protects the airway. Lesions in this area tend to present in advanced stages that cause symptoms related to swallowing difficulties (dysphagia) and aspiration.

The glottic area of the larynx is composed of the true vocal cords along with the anterior and posterior commissures. The vocal cords vibrate when air passes over them, resulting in phonation. The vocal cords also protect the airway during swallowing. Approximately 75% of all laryngeal tumors arise on the vocal cords (Bailey, 2001). Hoarseness for more than two weeks can be an early warning sign for tumors of the glottic larynx. Patients with cancer of the true vocal cord tend to present at an earlier stage because of early symptoms.

The subglottic area extends from the inferior edge of the true vocal cord to the lower border of the cricoid cartilage. Subglottic tumors are uncommon, and most tumors in this area are extensions of tumors originating in the supraglottic or glottic larynx (Bailey, 2001).

Before the 19th century, the treatment of laryngeal cancer, as well as that of most other laryngeal diseases, was limited almost exclusively to tracheotomy (Weir, 1990). This procedure was performed in cases of acute suffocation and was largely unsuccessful in decreasing morbidity and mortality. It was not until the late 19th century that physicians began to consider the removal of the entire larynx as a treatment for cancer. Austrian physician Theodore Bilroth performed the first total laryngectomy (TL) for the treatment of laryngeal cancer in 1873 and the first horizontal supraglottic laryngectomy (SGL) in 1883. Enrico Bottini of Italy is credited with performing the first TL with long-term patient survival in 1875. His patient was a young man with laryngeal sarcoma who lived for 10 years after the operation (Weir). Since that time, many advances and variations of Bilroth's original proce-

dures have been developed, including the hemilaryngectomy, SGL, supracricoid laryngectomy with cricohyoidopexy, and supracricoid laryngectomy with cricohyoidoepiglottopexy. These procedures, along with chemotherapy and radiotherapy, have allowed physicians to successfully treat many laryngeal cancers (Weir).

Early-stage laryngeal cancers usually are treated with radiation therapy, which achieves a high cure rate and an excellent functional outcome. Locally advanced laryngeal cancers often require a TL when treated surgically.

The Cooperative Studies Program of the Veterans Affairs Laryngeal Cancer Study Group focused on organ preservation in the treatment of advanced laryngeal cancer. This landmark study looked at survival rates of patients with locally advanced laryngeal cancer treated with chemotherapy and radiation and surgical salvage for nonresponders versus surgery (TL) and radiation. They found that the two-year survival rate for both groups was 68%. The larynx was preserved in 66% of the surviving patients or 31% of the entire group. At three years, 40% of the chemotherapy/radiation group were alive and disease free and had an intact larynx (Gopal, Frankenthaler, & Fried, 2001). Subsequent quality-of-life studies showed higher scores in the combined chemotherapy/radiation therapy group. The majority of patients with laryngeal cancer now are treated with radiation therapy or chemotherapy combined with radiation therapy. This trend toward organ preservation in patients with advanced laryngeal cancer leads to preservation of physiologic function and improved quality of life (Bailey, 2001).

Surgical management of laryngeal cancer is still important in the primary management of some patients and in the management of recurrent or persistent cancer after organ preservation therapy. This section will review surgical procedures commonly used in the treatment of laryngeal cancer: TL, SGL, vertical partial laryngectomy, and supracricoid laryngectomy with cricohyoidopexy. The indications, operative management, and anatomical considerations of each of these procedures will be discussed. Figure 6-7 shows the supraglottic, glottic, and subglottic levels of the larynx.

Supraglottic Laryngectomy

SGL is a horizontal resection of the upper part of the larynx. It is indicated for the treatment of T1, T2, and some T3 primary tumors of the supraglottic area. The area above the true vocal cords to the epiglottis is resected. This is indicated for cancers involving the laryngeal surface of the epiglottis, infrahyoid and suprahyoid epiglottis, ventricular folds, and aryepiglottic folds. Because most supraglottic tumors tend to remain confined above the glottis, the incision is made just above the vocal cords. The superior incision is usually at the level of the hyoid bone. If tumor extension is present, the SGL can be modified to include superior resection into the base of the tongue and inferior resection to include the glottis and

Figure 6-7. Levels of the Larynx

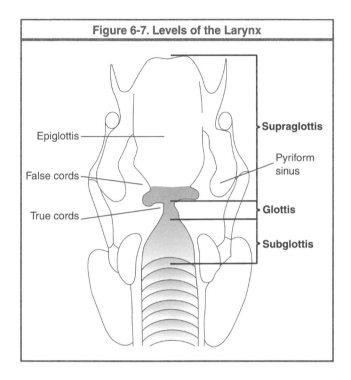

Epiglottis

False cords

True cords

Supraglottis

Pyriform sinus

Glottis

Subglottis

ment of primary supraglottic carcinomas (Silver & Ferlito, 1996). The most commonly encountered postoperative problem is aspiration of food because of resection of the epiglottis. This is the result of interruption of the sensory input of the swallowing mechanism. Cricopharyngeal myotomy is an incision through the cricopharyngeal muscle done at the time of initial resection or as a secondary procedure to minimize postoperative aspiration. Cricopharyngeal myotomy allows for relaxation of the sphincter during the second phase of swallowing. Other methods that prevent postoperative aspiration include suspension of the larynx and preservation of the internal laryngeal nerve (Silver & Ferlito).

Patients will need a referral to a speech-language specialist for swallowing and speech rehabilitation. They will be taught specific techniques to assist them in swallowing.

Supracricoid Laryngectomy With Cricohyoidopexy

Supracricoid laryngectomy with cricohyoidopexy (SCL-CHP) is a horizontal partial laryngeal surgical procedure that often allows patients with advanced supraglottic and transglottic cancers to safely avoid TL. The resection includes the entire supraglottis, the vocal cords, the entire thyroid cartilage, and up to one arytenoid cartilage. The reconstruction involves securing the cricoid to the hyoid bone. The result of the surgery is a hoarse but serviceable voice, maintenance of functional swallowing, and the ability to breathe without a permanent tracheotomy (Rassekh, Weinstein, & Laccourreye, 2001).

Indications for SCL-CHP are T2 and T3 supraglottic cancers that invade or extend into the glottic level, the anterior commissure, the floor of the ventricle, or the paraglottic space. Certain tumors with vocal cord fixation also may be treated with this procedure if some level of arytenoid function is present. The contraindications for SCL-CHP are invasions of the hyoid bone, preepiglottic space, valleculae, or tongue base. In addition, this procedure is contraindicated when the tumor has caused arytenoid fixation or with subglottic extension into the cricoid, pharyngeal or interarytenoid involvement, extensive thyroid cartilage invasion, or inadequate pulmonary reserve and when the tumor is resectable by SGL. Data on this procedure as an alternative to TL are promising. In a study by Laccourreye, Laccourreye, Weinstein, Menard, and Brasnu (1990), 95.4% of patients who underwent SCL-CHP recovered physiologic deglutition, and none required a permanent tracheotomy. No local recurrences were encountered, and the three-year survival rate was 71.4% (Laccourreye et al.). Although SCL-CHP often has been combined with irradiation for the treatment of glottic and supraglottic cancers, a study by Sessions et al. (2002) found no significant difference between patients who underwent conservative surgery (i.e., SCL-CHP) alone versus those who underwent conservative surgery combined with irradiation for T3N0M0 glottic carcinomas.

paraglottic space. Resection also can be extended laterally to include tumors of the pyriform sinus and posteriorly to include one arytenoid cartilage. Cure rates with conventional SGL are 70%–90% (DeSanto, 2001). SGL has been combined with radiation therapy both pre- and postoperatively. Edema of the remaining larynx can be a problem if the patient has been previously irradiated. A study by Yiotakis et al. (2003) found an increased morbidity in patients who underwent salvage SGL after irradiation failure, particularly in patients with T2 tumors. Contraindications for SGL are fixation or impaired motion of the true vocal cord, tumors within 5 mm of the anterior commissure, thyroid cartilage involvement, and underlying medical conditions, such as chronic pulmonary disease (one-second forced expiratory volume < 50%) or uncorrectable swallowing disorders.

Conventional SGL involves removal of the hyoid bone, the superior half of the thyroid cartilage, epiglottis, the false vocal cords, the aryepiglottic folds, and the ventricle. The neck dissection is the first step in the surgical procedure and typically is performed on the side of the neck containing the dominant portion of the lesion or the side with palpable lymph nodes. A bilateral neck dissection is recommended if biopsy from the first side of the neck is positive for metastasis. A modified neck dissection that preserves the internal jugular vein and accessory nerve is preferred (DeSanto, 2001).

SGL is preferred, when possible, over TL because the true vocal cords are preserved, allowing for the maintenance of laryngeal function. Patients will have a temporary tracheotomy until postoperative edema of the surgical site resolves. Cure rates for SGL consistently range from 70%–80% in the treat-

Partial Laryngectomy

Partial laryngectomy refers to a group of surgical procedures that includes cordectomy, vertical partial laryngectomy, or other type of hemilaryngectomy. Open cordectomy (as opposed to endoscopic cordectomy) is limited to lesions confined to the true vocal cord. In each of these procedures, the larynx is exposed through a neck incision and the tumor is visualized (Bailey, 2001).

The cordectomy consists of a limited excision of the true vocal cord with exposure accomplished by a midline thyrotomy (incision through the thyroid cartilage). This procedure is indicated when the lesion does not extend to the anterior commissure or involve the arytenoid cartilage. The vertical partial laryngectomy or other form of hemilaryngectomy is performed when the tumor involves the anterior commissure or the lesion extends into the vocal process of the arytenoids. It also is performed on superficial transglottic lesions and on areas of recurrence after radiation therapy (Bailey, 2001). Partial laryngectomy is not indicated when the tumor extends to the posterior commissure, where the tumor invades the thyroid cartilage or arytenoid cartilage on both sides, or with a vocal cord that is fixed because of tumor involvement (Bailey).

Tracheotomy is performed to maintain a patent airway because of postoperative edema. Edema that persists for more than six to eight weeks may indicate a tumor and should be assessed. Patients who received radiation therapy before surgery are at increased risk for edema. Patients will need a referral to a speech-language specialist for swallowing and speech rehabilitation.

Total Laryngectomy

Even with the advent of more conservative surgical techniques, TL remains the standard by which all other treatments for laryngeal cancer are measured. TL still is commonly performed in the treatment of advanced cancers of the larynx, especially for salvage surgery after irradiation failure. It also is performed in conjunction with removal of the entire hypopharynx for surgical management of hypopharyngeal tumors.

TL involves removal of the entire larynx, including the thyroid and cricoid cartilages as well as the hyoid bone. A permanent opening for breathing, or stoma, is created by suturing the trachea to the skin of the anterior neck. Air can no longer enter the upper aerodigestive tract of the patient following TL (see Figure 6-8). This results in a loss of the sense of smell, which, in turn, diminishes the sense of taste. Patients can no longer sneeze, sniff, or blow the nose. TL is indicated for stage III and IV carcinomas of the larynx or stage II cancers unsuitable for partial laryngectomy. TL also is indicated for subglottic or glottic carcinomas with subglottic extension of more than 1.5 cm, for carcinoma of the base of the tongue extending beyond the circumvallate papillae that invades into the larynx, and for failed radiotherapy for

Figure 6-8. Anatomy Changes Before and After Laryngectomy

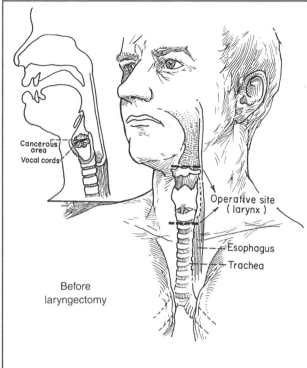

Before laryngectomy

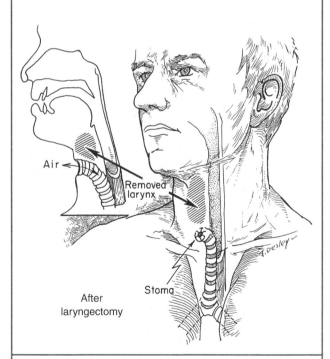

After laryngectomy

Note. From *Looking Forward: A Guidebook for the Laryngectomee* (3rd ed., pp. 8–9), by R.L. Keith, 1995, New York: Thieme New York. Copyright 1995 by Thieme New York. Reprinted with permission.

laryngeal carcinoma. It is contraindicated in elderly patients with distant metastases and in patients with poor medical status (Gopal et al., 2001).

TL is a radical procedure that may be combined with postoperative radiation in advanced cases. In a recent series of 628 patients with T4 cancer of the larynx treated with TL and postoperative radiation, the overall actuarial and disease-free survival rates at seven years were 43% and 30%, respectively (Ampil et al., 2004).

Voice rehabilitation is an essential part of the postoperative management of TL patients. Various options are available to rehabilitate the voice, including developing esophageal speech, using a tracheoesophageal voice prosthesis, or using an electrolarynx. Esophageal speech is produced by compressing air into the esophagus and then releasing it in a controlled fashion. This results in vibratory movement of the pharyngeal-esophageal segment. This method is difficult to learn and often produces an undesirable type of voice. Esophageal speech largely has been replaced by tracheoesophageal puncture (TEP), in which a prosthesis is inserted into a surgically created tracheoesophageal fistula. Pulmonary air is diverted through a one-way valve in the device, causing vibration of the pharyngeal-esophageal segment and voice production. This procedure provides superior voice intelligibility when compared to any other method of rehabilitation (Beasley & Gullane, 2003). The TEP procedure can be performed at the time of TL or as a separate procedure after any postoperative treatment.

When the surgical resection includes removal of a portion of the pharynx with TL, reconstruction with a pedicled or microvascular free flap usually is required. Partial pharyngectomy defects can be reconstructed with a pedicled pectoralis major myocutaneous flap or a microvascular free flap, such as a radial forearm fasciocutaneous flap. Circumferential pharyngectomy defects are best reconstructed with a jejunal microvascular free flap or, occasionally, a gastric pull-up.

Maxillectomy

Malignancies of the sinonasal tract characterize less than 1% of all malignant tumors and almost 3% of all tumors in the upper respiratory tract. The incidence in males is twice that of females and is more common in white males 50–70 years of age. Individuals who work in industries with exposure to wood dust, the tanning of leather, and the nickel refining process are at increased risk for development of these tumors. The most common site for malignant tumors of the sinonasal tract is the maxillary sinus. Squamous cell carcinoma is the most common malignancy in the sinonasal tract; however, adenocarcinoma also is found in the ethmoid sinus and nasal cavity. Adenocarcinoma comprises up to 8% of tumors found in the sinonasal tract (Carrau & Myers, 2001).

Since its conception in the mid-19th century, the maxillectomy has been the standard surgical procedure for

the treatment of advanced maxillary sinus cancer. French physician Joseph Gensoul performed the first total maxillectomy in 1827, without anesthesia, on a patient with a large osteosarcoma. In 1941, British physician Robert Liston performed a radical maxillectomy on a 21-year-old man with an angiofibroma at University College Hospital in London (Weir, 1990). Throughout the 19th and 20th centuries, many advances were made in the technique and approach to tumors of the maxillary sinus.

Enormous diversity exists in the histology, site of origin, and behavior of tumors treated by maxillectomy. A study of 403 maxillectomies reported 29 different histologic diagnoses, including squamous cell carcinoma, sarcoma, melanoma, malignant fibro-osseous lesions, and benign mucosal lesions (Spiro, Strong, & Shah, 1997). With this diversity of pathology comes several variations on the maxillectomy, including medial maxillectomy, the Weber-Fergusson approach to total and subtotal maxillectomy, total maxillectomy with orbital preservation, and total maxillectomy with orbital exenteration.

This section will review the indications and operative management for a radical maxillectomy with orbital exenteration. Conservative variations on this procedure will be discussed with reference to the total maxillectomy.

Total Maxillectomy With Orbital Exenteration

Total maxillectomy with orbital exenteration is an *en bloc* resection of the maxilla, including dental structures, ethmoid labyrinth, anterior zygoma, and the orbit and adnexal structures. It is indicated for malignant tumors of the maxillary sinus or maxilla with superior extension into the orbit. Total maxillectomy with orbital exenteration also may be indicated for aggressive infection of the maxillary sinuses in immunocompromised patients. Pathways of invasion leading from the maxillary sinus to the orbit include direct bony extension, perivascular or perineural invasion by way of the infraorbital or ethmoidial neurovascular bundles, or the infraorbital fissure or nasolacrimal duct (Carrau & Myers, 2001). Survival rates for patients who have advanced disease requiring orbital exenteration are poor. This leads surgeons to perform this procedure only when there is orbital wall involvement at the time of surgery (Nazar, Rodrigo, Llorente, Baragano, & Suarez, 2004).

The defects associated with total maxillectomy with orbital exenteration include the loss of smell (which affects taste), loss of vision, cosmetic facial deformity, facial numbness and paralysis, and difficulty with swallowing and speech. Reconstruction and rehabilitation are accomplished with flaps, grafts, and prosthodontic devices.

Surgical defects created by a total maxillectomy with orbital exenteration will require a flap that has substantial muscle and skin to reconstruct the resected area. In some cases, bone is used to reconstruct the orbital rim and floor. Various microvascular myocutaneous free flaps, including latissimus dorsi, rectus abdominus, and scapular fasciocutaneous flap, can be used. The goals of flap reconstruction are to promote primary wound healing, reestablish the facial contour, create oronasal separation, and separate the cranial cavity from the upper aerodigestive tract if the skull base has been resected. Flap reconstruction can facilitate speech and swallowing rehabilitation (Bailey, 2001).

A split thickness skin graft (STSG) is placed over exposed areas. Packing or a bolster may be inserted intraoperatively and secured over the STSG to ensure adherence to the exposed areas of the undersurface of the cheek flap. The bolster temporarily fills the surgical defect, allowing the patient to speak and swallow after surgery. The bolster is removed five to seven days postoperatively.

A prosthetic device known as a palatal obturator also may be used. It is prepared preoperatively and resembles an upper denture. This device is wired to any remaining dentition or to the hard palate at the time of resection. It holds packing in place and allows for swallowing and intelligible speech during the postoperative phase. Once the packing is removed, additional material is applied to the obturator to fill in the surgical defect. Refinements are made postoperatively as healing occurs and edema subsides. The obturator must fit properly to provide for swallowing and speech and should be easily removed for cleaning (see Figure 6-9).

for the removal of lesions limited to the anterior nasal cavity and adjacent medial third of the maxillary and ethmoid sinuses (Knudsen & Bailey, 2001). Lateral rhinotomy is used for *en bloc* resections of the ethmoid labyrinth and the wall between the antrum and nasal cavity when infiltrated by tumor (Lawson & Biller, 1991).

The lateral rhinotomy incision is made along the side of the nose. This incision extends from the nostril around the alar groove, up the side of the nose, over the upper lateral cartilage, and around the frontal process of the maxilla to the medial canthus and the medial end of the eyebrow. The incision should be made within natural creases of the skin to prevent cosmetic deformity. The incision is made to the depth of the periosteum of the bone. To provide more access to the antrum, the incision can be extended at its lower end to split the upper lip. It also can be extended further to form a full-face flap for maxillectomy or into the upper eyelid for exenteration of the orbital contents. The basic incision contains the flexibility needed for all sinus and nasal operations (Neel & Fee, 1998) (see Figure 6-10).

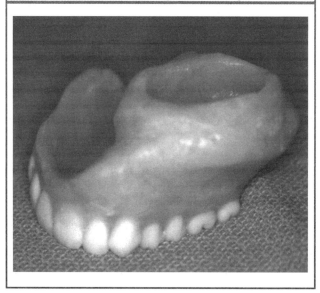

Figure 6-9. Prosthetic Obturator for Patient Following Maxillectomy

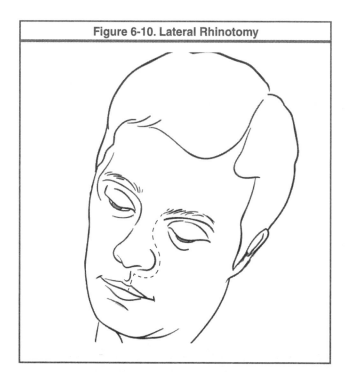

Figure 6-10. Lateral Rhinotomy

Lateral Rhinotomy

The lateral rhinotomy is a surgical incision that provides access to the nasal cavity through the lateral wall. A lateral rhinotomy is indicated for surgical access to the nasal cavity, paranasal sinuses, and nasopharynx. It is a useful approach

Mandibulectomy

The oral cavity is composed of the lips, tongue, buccal mucosa, FOM, hard palate, and alveolar ridges. The area of transition to the oropharynx is the retromolar trigone (see Figure 2-6). This area is located behind the third molar next to the FOM and anterior to the tonsillar pillar and soft palate. Known as the "coffin corner," this area can harbor lesions that are quite small and can be easily missed on examination. The lesions can remain hidden until they become large enough to be symptomatic (Donald, 1984).

The management of primary tumors of the oral cavity may include surgical excision, radiotherapy, chemotherapy, or a combination of these modalities. Radiation and surgical excision are equally successful in treating early-stage tumors in this area. Each of these modalities has advantages and disadvantages. Radiation therapy allows for avoidance of surgery and anesthesia and their associated risks. However, significant side effects include xerostomia, dysgeusia, and the need for full-mouth teeth extraction. The surgical option allows for rapid rehabilitation of the patient and avoidance of radiation side effects. However, the major disadvantages are functional disability and cosmetic defect, depending on the size of the resection (Sharma, Schuller, & Baker, 1998).

Surgery is preferred over radiation in patients who continue to smoke and drink alcohol excessively because they are at high risk for developing other primary tumors in this area. Surgical resection in combination with radiotherapy is preferred for advanced tumors of the oral cavity, especially when they have invaded into the mandible or the mandibular periosteum (Sharma et al., 1998). Lesions that have infiltrated bone or that extend close to the mandible (where a 2-cm margin of tumor-free tissue is not possible with resection of the primary lesion) require resection of the involved mandible in addition to the involved part of the oral cavity (Myers, 2001). Several studies have demonstrated reduced rates of local recurrence and improved survival rates in patients with advanced malignancies undergoing combined surgery and radiation therapy (Carvalho, Ikeda, Magrin, & Kowalski, 2004; Sharma et al.). Chemotherapy as an adjuvant to surgery and radiation is an area of active investigation (Sharma et al.).

Segmental Mandibulectomy

Segmental mandibulectomy is indicated for primary benign or malignant neoplasms of the mandible and for tumors that have invaded the mandible from adjacent tissue. Segmental mandibulectomy is contraindicated when the tumor can be treated with a marginal approach and for tumors (i.e., lymphomas, distant metastases) that are more appropriately treated with radiation therapy or chemotherapy.

A tracheotomy is performed to ensure a stable airway and to provide better intraoral exposure. A lip splitting incision or a visor flap incision then is performed. The skin flap is elevated, carefully ensuring the integrity of the marginal mandibular nerve. If the tumor is malignant, the mandibular bone is resected *en bloc* with surrounding soft tissue. Surgical margins of grossly normal mandibles of 1–1.5 cm are appropriate. A frozen section of the inferior alveolar nerve then is obtained. Because there is no reliable method of assessing bony tumor extension intraoperatively, and if sections of the inferior alveolar nerve are positive for tumor, the entire inferior alveolar canal is resected.

Reconstruction of a segmental mandibular resection is recommended in all patients, but the type of reconstruction depends on the specific case. Lateral defects (in edentulous patients) posterior to the angle of the mandible do well with soft-tissue closure or closure with a pedicled myocutaneous flap. Defects of the anterior arch of the mandible should undergo immediate reconstruction of the mandible with a bone-containing flap. The microvascular osteomyocutaneous flap provides excellent reconstruction of the bony mandible and associated soft tissues.

Two common osteomyocutaneous flaps used in this area are the fibular free flap and the iliac crest free flap. The fibular free flap is used when bone is needed but there is minimal need for soft-tissue reconstruction. The fibula is a straight bone that has a very rich blood supply. A length of approximately 25 cm can be harvested with minimal donor site complications. Because of the rich blood supply, multiple osteotomies (cuts in the bone) can be made to allow the bone to be contoured as needed. Muscle, tissue, and skin that are harvested with the fibula can be used to reconstruct soft tissue defects that were created at the time of resection. Osseointegrated implants can be used with this type of reconstruction to provide dental restoration after adequate healing has occurred (Levine & Hood, 2001). This type of reconstruction optimally addresses both functional and cosmetic concerns related to resection of the mandible.

The iliac crest free flap is another type of osteomyocutaneous flap used for reconstruction. The natural shape of the iliac crest allows it to conform to the mandible with fewer osteotomies. The blood supply to the skin pedicle in this type of flap is poor, thus requiring a larger skin pedicle to include more blood vessels, giving the flap a bulky soft tissue component with little mobility. The iliac crest flap is used for reconstruction that requires a large amount of soft tissue (i.e., those found in large craniofacial defects) (Levine & Hood, 2001). It is not used frequently because of its excessive bulk, which results in decreased function, a short vascular pedicle, significant donor site morbidity, and less cosmetic appeal because of skin color differences.

An alternative to a free flap reconstruction, especially when the patient is not a candidate for a free flap, is a mandibular reconstructive plate with a pectoralis major pedicle flap (Myers, 2001). This approach provides adequate reconstruction and closure to the wound; however, cosmetic and functional deficiencies to the chest and neck are common. This flap has considerable bulk, resulting in a prominence in the neck that can be cosmetically unappealing and can restrict range of motion to the neck. This approach is not used for defects of the anterior mandibular arch.

The free flap procedures require microvascular surgical expertise and an increase in operative time. Candidates for these types of reconstructive procedures must be considered carefully. Underlying medical conditions, such as cardiovascular disease, diabetes mellitus, poor nutritional status, and continued use of tobacco, may compromise vascularity and thus jeopardize viability of these flaps. Successful outcomes depend on careful preoperative assessment and a well-coordinated multidisciplinary approach to treatment.

Glossectomy

Cancer of the tongue constitutes 20%–50% of all oral cavity carcinomas. Carcinoma of the oral tongue most commonly arises from the lateral border of the middle third of the tongue; approximately 45% of all tongue cancers occur here. In contrast, 20% of cancers occur in the anterior third and only 4% on the dorsum of the tongue (Sharma et al., 1998). Several treatment options are available, depending on the extent of the tumor.

Partial Glossectomy

Partial glossectomy is indicated for T1, T2, and T3 lesions that are limited to the anterior two-thirds of the tongue. Resection of the lesion with primary closure results in minimal loss of function to speech and swallowing. If the FOM is involved, the area is resected and reconstructed with an STSG (Sharma et al., 1998). This will allow mobility of the remaining tongue and reconstructs the FOM. Large defects that cannot be closed primarily or communicate with the neck often are reconstructed with microvascular free tissue flaps, most commonly a radial forearm fasciocutaneous flap. This flap provides a barrier between the oral cavity and the neck, preventing wound breakdown and fistula formation. Most T1 and smaller T2 lesions of the anterior tongue can be treated successfully with surgery alone. Larger lesions or smaller lesions with aggressive features often are treated with surgery and postoperative radiation therapy. Base-of-tongue (posterior one-third of the tongue) cancers can be treated with either surgery or radiation therapy. Many of these lesions are treated with radiation therapy or chemotherapy because of functional defects associated with the surgery.

Controversy exists concerning elective treatment of the neck for early-stage tongue lesions with no palpable lymph node metastasis. Despite any survival benefit, a staging neck dissection often is performed for all but the most superficial T1 lesions. Even if the tongue lesion is in an early stage, patients with lymph node metastases in the neck generally will require postoperative radiation therapy. Treatment for stage III and IV disease requires combined modalities to better control local and regional disease (Johnson, 1996).

Total Glossectomy

The need for total glossectomy depends on the invasion of the tumor into the substance of the tongue as well as involvement of the neurovascular supply to the tongue. Total glossectomy is indicated for massive tumors of the oral tongue, tumors involving both sides of the base of the tongue, and large tumors of the FOM involving the ventral surface of the tongue or extending deeply in the FOM to involve the submental area (Kraus & Joe, 2003). A tracheotomy is done for airway maintenance at the beginning of the procedure. A bilateral SND is performed for the node-negative (N0) neck, or an MRND is performed on patients with palpable adenopathy. Defects resulting from total glossectomy are reconstructed with a pectoralis major myocutaneous flap that reinforces the wound circumferentially. Suction drains are placed along the region of the reconstruction bilaterally (Johnson, 1996).

Historically, patients who had a total glossectomy also had a TL to prevent intractable aspiration pneumonia. With modern reconstructive techniques, retention of the larynx can be considered in medically stable patients who are motivated to attempt to relearn swallowing. After total glossectomy, the patient has no separation between the oral and pharyngeal phases of swallowing. The mouth acts as a passive conduit because the lack of a tongue eliminates the ability to control and propel the bolus into the posterior oral cavity. Feeding is performed using a syringe and liquid diet that can be directed into the posterior oral cavity. After a total glossectomy, speech may be intelligible to family members and close acquaintances. Deficits in articulation occur because of the lack of a mobile tongue (Kraus & Joe, 2003).

Summary

This review has outlined some of the common types of surgeries performed in the management of head and neck malignancies. The challenges to management and treatment of head and neck cancers are significant. No other type of malignancy is so visible to the public. To remove the malignancy and maintain and restore function along with preserving cosmetic appearance still remains a challenge. Head and neck cancers are among the most debilitating malignancies because they affect basic functioning, such as the ability to breathe, speak, and eat (Scarpa, 2004). Optimal care of these patients requires active, intense support following the acute surgical intervention and discharge to an outpatient setting. This support includes assistance in maintaining an adequate airway and nutritional status as well as developing ways of communicating. Patients with head and neck cancer often are faced with the challenge of caring for tubes for breathing (tracheostomy tubes) and for feeding (gastrostomy tubes and nasogastric tubes). Their ability to ambulate and communicate often is impaired (Scarpa).

The quality of life and the very survival of these patients are directly dependent on their ability to become self-sufficient in certain areas of their care and to receive assistance from individuals able to cope with the demands of caring for them. A coordinated multidisciplinary approach utilizing the hospital, community, and family resources can provide optimal care and survival for patients with head and neck cancer (Scarpa, 2004).

References

Ampil, F., Nathan, C.A., Caldito, G., Lian, T.F., Aarstad, R.F., & Krishnamsetty, R.M. (2004). Total laryngectomy and postoperative radiotherapy for T4 laryngeal cancer: A 14-year review. *American Journal of Otolaryngology, 25,* 88–93.

Bailey, B.J. (2001). Vertical partial laryngectomy and laryngoplasty. In B.J. Bailey (Ed.), *Head and neck surgery—Otolaryngology* (3rd ed., pp. 1469–1482). Philadelphia: Lippincott Williams and Wilkins.

Beasley, N., & Gullane, P. (2003). Cancer of the larynx, paranasal sinuses, and temporal bone. In K.J. Lee (Ed.), *Essential otolaryngology: Head and neck surgery* (8th ed., pp. 596–616). New York: McGraw-Hill.

Carrau, R., & Myers, E.N. (2001). Neoplasms of the nose and paranasal sinuses. In B.J. Bailey (Ed.), *Head and neck surgery—Otolaryngology* (3rd ed., pp. 1247–1266). Philadelphia: Lippincott Williams and Wilkins.

Carvalho, A.L., Ikeda, M.K., Magrin, J., & Kowalski, L.P. (2004). Trends of oral and oropharyngeal cancer survival over five decades in 3267 patients treated in a single institution. *Oral Oncology, 40,* 71–76.

Crile, G. (1987). Landmark article Dec. 1, 1906: Excision of cancer of the head and neck. With special reference to the plan of dissection based on one hundred and thirty-two operations. *JAMA, 258,* 3286–3293.

DeSanto, L.W. (2001). Supraglottic laryngectomy. In B.J. Bailey (Ed.), *Head and neck surgery—Otolaryngology* (3rd ed., pp. 1483–1494). Philadelphia: Lippincott Williams and Wilkins.

Donald, P.J. (1984). *Head and neck cancer: Management of the difficult case.* Philadelphia: W.B. Saunders.

Dubner, S. (2004, August 19). *Head and neck cancer: Resection and neck dissection.* Retrieved November 29, 2004, from http://www.emedicine.com/plastic/topic370.htm

Gopal, H., Frankenthaler, R., & Fried, M.P. (2001). Advanced cancer of the larynx. In B.J. Bailey (Ed.), *Head and neck surgery—Otolaryngology* (3rd ed., pp. 1505–1522). Philadelphia: Lippincott Williams and Wilkins.

Johnson, J.T. (1996). Total glossectomy. In B.J. Bailey (Ed.), *Atlas of head and neck surgery—Otolaryngology* (pp. 82–83). Philadelphia: Lippincott Williams and Wilkins.

Knudsen, S.J., & Bailey, B.J. (2001). Midline nasal masses. In B.J. Bailey (Ed.), *Head and neck surgery—Otolaryngology* (3rd ed., pp. 309–320). Philadelphia: Lippincott Williams and Wilkins.

Kraus, D.H., & Joe, J.K. (2003). Neoplasms of the oral cavity and oropharynx. In J.B. Snow & J.J. Ballenger (Eds.), *Ballenger's otorhinolaryngology: Head and neck surgery* (16th ed., pp. 1408–1436). Hamilton, Ontario, Canada: B.C. Decker.

Laccourreye, H., Laccourreye, O., Weinstein, G., Menard, M., & Brasnu, D. (1990). Supracricoid laryngectomy with cricohyoidopexy: A partial laryngeal procedure for selected supraglottic and transglottic carcinomas. *Laryngoscope, 100,* 735–741.

Lawson, W., & Biller, H.F. (1991). Lateral rhinotomy. In A. Blitzer, W. Lawson, & W. Friedman (Eds.), *Surgery of the paranasal sinuses* (2nd ed., pp. 297–308). Philadelphia: W.B. Saunders.

Levine, P.A., & Hood, R.J. (2001). Neoplasms of the oral cavity. In B.J. Bailey (Ed.), *Head and neck surgery—Otolaryngology* (3rd ed., pp. 1311–1326). Philadelphia: Lippincott Williams and Wilkins.

Muller, C.D., Newlands, S., Quinn, F.B., & Ryan, M.W. (2002, January 16). *Neck dissection: Classification, indications and techniques.* Paper presented at the University of Texas Medical Branch Grand Rounds on January 16, 2002. Retrieved August 5, 2003, from http://www.utmb.edu/otoref/Grnds/Neck-Dissection-020116/Neck-Dissection-020116.htm

Myers, E.N. (2001). Floor of mouth resection with lateral mandible invasion. In B.J. Bailey (Ed.), *Atlas of head and neck surgery—Otolaryngology* (pp. 90–91). Philadelphia: Lippincott Williams and Wilkins.

Nazar, G., Rodrigo, J.P., Llorente, J.L., Baragano, L., & Suarez, C. (2004). Prognostic factors of maxillary sinus malignancies. *American Journal of Rhinology, 18,* 233–238.

Neel, H.B., III, & Fee, W.E., Jr. (1998). Benign and malignant tumors of the nasopharynx. In C.W. Cummings, J.M. Fredrickson, C.A. Harker, C.J. Krause, M.A. Richardson, & D.E. Schuller (Eds.), *Otolaryngology: Head and neck surgery* (3rd ed., pp. 1512–1526). St. Louis, MO: Mosby.

Rassekh, C.H., Weinstein, G.S., & Laccourreye, O. (2001). Supracricoid partial laryngectomy. In B.J. Bailey (Ed.), *Head and neck surgery—Otolaryngology* (3rd ed., pp. 1495–1504). Philadelphia: Lippincott Williams and Wilkins.

Robbins, K.T. (2001). *Pocket guide to neck dissection classification and TNM staging of head and neck cancer* (2nd ed.). Alexandria, VA: American Academy of Otolaryngology—Head and Neck Surgery Foundation.

Robbins, K.T., Clayman, G., Levine, P.A., Medina, J., Sessions, R., Shaha, A., et al. (2002). Neck dissection classification update: Revisions proposed by the American Head and Neck Society and American Academy of Otolaryngology—Head and Neck Surgery. *Archives of Otolaryngology—Head and Neck Surgery, 128,* 751–758.

Robbins, K.T., Medina, J.E., Wolfe, G.T., Levine, P.A., Sessions, R.B., & Pruet, C.W. (1991). Standardizing neck dissection terminology: Official report of the Academy's Committee for Head and Neck Surgery and Oncology. *Archives of Otolaryngology—Head & Neck Surgery, 117,* 601–605.

Scarpa, R. (2004). Advanced practice nursing in head and neck cancer: Application of the five behaviors. *Oncology Nursing Forum, 31,* 579–583.

Sessions, D.G., Lenox, J., Spector, G.J., Newland, D., Simpson, J., Haughey, B., et al. (2002). Management of T3N0M0 glottic carcinoma: Therapeutic outcomes. *Laryngoscope, 112,* 1281–1288.

Shah, J.P., & Patel, S.G. (2003). *Head and neck surgery and oncology* (3rd ed., pp. 353–395). St. Louis, MO: Mosby.

Sharma, P.K., Schuller, D.E., & Baker, S.R. (1998). Malignant neoplasms of the oral cavity. In C.W. Cummings, J.M. Fredrickson, C.A. Harker, C.J. Krause, M.A. Richardson, & D.E. Schuller (Eds.), *Otolaryngology—Head and neck surgery* (3rd ed., pp. 1430–1443). St. Louis, MO: Mosby.

Silver, C.E., & Ferlito, A. (1996). *Surgery for cancer of the larynx and related structures* (2nd ed.). Philadelphia: W.B. Saunders.

Spiro, R.H., Strong, E.W., & Shah, J.P. (1997). Maxillectomy and its classification. *Head and Neck, 19,* 309–314.

Weir, N. (1990). *Otolaryngology: An illustrated history.* London: Butterworths.

Yiotakis, J., Stavroulaki, P., Nikolopoulos, T., Manolopoulos, L., Kandiloros, D., Ferekidis, E., et al. (2003). Partial laryngectomy after irradiation failure. *Otolaryngology—Head and Neck Surgery, 128,* 200–209.

CHAPTER 7

Radiation Treatment and Symptom Management

Lisa L. Blevins, RN, BSN, OCN®

Introduction

Radiation therapy (RT) plays an important role in the management of head and neck cancer. Radiation may be used as a primary treatment for small tumors (stages I and II), as adjuvant treatment for larger tumors (stages III and IV), or as a palliative measure for patients with unresectable or recurrent tumors. RT may be given alone or in combination with surgery and/or chemotherapy to provide better local-regional tumor control. RT alone is the most common treatment for certain types and stages of head and neck cancer, such as cancer of the nasopharynx, larynx, and oropharynx (Hoffman, Karnell, Funk, Robinson, & Menck, 1998; Rose-Ped et al., 2002). The principal goal of RT is to eradicate or control tumor cells while minimizing toxicity to the surrounding normal tissues (Boelsen & Jamar, 2000). RT also can be given to achieve cure. If a cure is not realistic, RT can be given to control the progression of disease. Finally, RT can be given during the terminal stage of cancer for palliative relief of pain caused by bone metastasis, obstruction caused by tumor progression, or uncontrolled bleeding resulting from tumor invasion of the vascular system.

Advances in technology combined with the effects of radiobiology have led to sophisticated treatment approaches, but these treatments can result in both acute and late sequelae. Consequently, patients with head and neck cancer need to receive care from a multidisciplinary team whose members can provide prospective treatment recommendations and support (Chou, Wilder, Wong, & Forster, 2001).

Principles of Treatment

RT is the treatment of cancer using ionizing radiation (electromagnetic energy) with very short wave lengths and very high energy intensity. Radiation is either electromagnetic or particulate and causes ionization within the cell (Holland, 2002). Ionizing radiation has sufficient energy to eject one or more orbital electrons from an atom or molecule, changing a stable atom to an ionized, unstable atom. Ionizing radiation interacts with tissues to create physical-chemical-biologic changes (Sitton, 1998). These biologic changes occur at the cellular level, where cell damage is both direct and indirect. Direct effects are accomplished by damage to critical molecules, such as DNA. When DNA is damaged, cell death or mutation may occur. Indirectly, radiation affects the water molecules surrounding the cell, resulting in biologic damage. Cell death takes place during the mitotic phase of the cell cycle, and the damaged cell is no longer able to reproduce.

Radiobiology

Radiobiology examines the effects of ionizing radiation on living organisms. Radiobiology has four central concepts: repair, repopulation, reassortment, and reoxygenation. Repair is the ability of normal tissues as well as cancer tissues to repair damage within 4–24 hours after radiation is delivered. As treatment progresses, tumor cells become less capable of repair. Repopulation or regeneration of healthy cells continues after repair of sublethal injury, allowing mitosis to take place. Tumor cells are more likely to die during mitosis. Redistribution of tumor cells in these cycles enhances the effectiveness of each succeeding radiation dose because more cells are likely to be in mitosis at the same time and healthy cells are less likely to redistribute (Hilderley, 1997). Reoxygenation occurs when well-oxygenated tumor cells die between daily doses, creating an environment in which previously hypoxic cells are exposed to capillary oxygenation. This reoxygenation effectively increases the success of the radiation treatments by increasing cell kill during subsequent doses (Boelsen & Jamar, 2000).

Fractionation

External beam radiation is prescribed by a radiation oncologist to deliver a total dose of ionized radiation to a tumor site.

This total dose is divided into smaller daily doses called fractions. Fractionation allows for reoxygenation of tumor cells as they become exposed to improved circulation, enhancing their radiosensitivity (Holland, 2002). The dose of radiation is expressed in units of gray (Gy), centigray (cGy), and radiation-absorbed dose (RAD) (1 Gy = 100 cGy = 100 RAD). In general, 44–50 Gy of radiation, delivered in increments of 1.8–2.0 Gy per fraction, are administered to regions that have a risk of 15% or more of harboring microscopic disease (Chou et al., 2001). Typically, 66–70 Gy are prescribed for primary tumors measuring 2 cm or less. When a patient with a more advanced disease receives RT alone, doses of 70 Gy or more are necessary to control the primary tumor and involved lymph nodes (Chou et al.). The goal of fractionation is to deliver a dose of radiation sufficient to kill the tumor while allowing the nearby normal tissues time to repair. A standard fractionation schedule is delivered five days a week for six to eight weeks of therapy.

Altered Fractionation

Locoregional control in advanced head and neck cancer is suboptimal when RT alone is administered on a once-daily schedule. For radiobiologic reasons, altered fractionation schedules in which two or three doses of radiation are delivered daily (at least six hours apart to minimize toxicity) have been studied in the treatment of advanced head and neck cancers (Chou et al., 2001). Hyperfractionation refers to twice-daily RT delivery. Higher daily doses can be given by administering two smaller dose treatments six hours apart. Instead of administering 1.8 Gy a day, 2.5 Gy can be delivered in two treatments of 1.25 Gy each. Accelerated fractionation uses a total dose and fraction size similar to conventional treatment but achieves a shorter overall treatment time by giving two to three doses daily. Accelerated hyperfractionation incorporates features of both accelerated fractionation and hyperfractionation. This hybrid regimen has been studied as a way of increasing tumor kill without increasing the risk of late complications (Chou et al.). Concomitant boost technique is a regimen that delivers once-daily treatments for the first 3.5 weeks and then twice daily during the final 2–2.5 weeks (Chou et al.). A final approach to the treatment schedule is hypofractionation, most commonly defined as administration of fewer than five fractionations per week. This schedule can deliver higher doses of treatment (e.g., 6.0 Gy on Mondays and Thursdays only). Hypofractionation has been used to deliver RT to a head and neck region after resection of cutaneous melanoma (Ang et al., 1994).

Chemotherapy

A number of antineoplastic agents appear to have radiosensitizing properties. The term *radiosensitizer* refers to compounds that enhance the damaging effects of ionizing radiation. Chemotherapy combined with RT as primary treatment for advanced head and neck cancers has become more prominent in recent years. Based on the findings of Al-Sarraf (2002), the standard of care for stage III or IV nasopharyngeal carcinoma is considered to be RT with concurrent cisplatin followed by 5-fluorouracil and cisplatin. Brizel et al. (2000) reported results of a randomized trial wherein the outcome of twice-daily RT and concurrent 5-fluorouracil and cisplatin chemotherapy was superior to that of twice-daily RT alone. The acute toxicities of chemotherapy with RT can be much more severe than either therapy alone.

Radiation Therapy Delivery Techniques

External Beam

External beam radiation therapy (EBRT), or teletherapy, is the delivery of local treatment by a linear accelerator. The linear accelerator can deliver treatment by high-energy x-rays (photons), gamma rays, or electrons. High-energy x-ray beams can penetrate intermediate to deep tissue depths, depending on the energy level used. Electron beam therapy delivers a shallow treatment and spares deeper tissues. Photon and electron beams often are used together to treat head and neck cancers. The high-energy x-rays are the primary treatment, and the electrons boost (i.e., give extra radiation dose) superficial tissues at the tumor site.

Traditional radiation planning is performed in two dimensions. An external contour of the patient's treatment area is traced on paper and digitized into a computer. X-ray films are taken of the area to be treated, and the radiation oncologist draws the anatomy on the film. These data are then combined to determine the treatment plan (Boelsen & Jamar, 2000).

Three-Dimensional Conformal Radiotherapy

Three-dimensional conformal radiotherapy (3DCRT) began in the late 1980s and early 1990s, allowing more precise delivery of the radiation dose. 3DCRT uses three-dimensional diagnostic images and computerized treatment programs to target the tumor from several angles (Berkowitz & Malin, 2002). 3DCRT has increased the accuracy of treatments; therefore, higher doses can be delivered to tumors with less damage to critical normal tissues (Boelsen & Jamar, 2000).

Both traditional and 3DCRT use custom-molded Cerrobend® (Cerro Metal Products, Bellefonte, PA) or lead blocks to shape the radiation beam. A different block is used for each treatment angle. These blocks are mounted on the linear accelerator by hand, which is slow and labor intensive (Berkowitz & Malin, 2002). Multileaf collimator (MLC) is a computer-controlled treatment shaping system. The radiation beam can now be automatically shaped by up to 120 individually controlled leaves housed inside the linear accelerator

(Berkowitz & Malin). This allows 3DCRT to be given more accurately and quickly.

Intensity-Modulated Radiation Therapy

Intensity-modulated radiation therapy (IMRT) is the latest technologic advance in EBRT. IMRT can deliver radiation more conformally than 3DCRT. IMRT differs from 3DCRT in that each x-ray beam is broken up into many "beamlets," and the intensity of each beamlet can be adjusted individually (Chou et al., 2001). The adjustable leaves of the MLC control not only the shape of the beam but also the exposure duration for each segment of the tumor, effectively modulating the dose within the treatment volume (Berkowitz & Malin, 2002). IMRT especially is useful in treating tumors of the nasal cavity, ethmoid and sphenoid sinuses, and base of the skull—areas where the risks of optic neuropathy and retinopathy following conventional RT are high (Chou et al.). Stereotactic radiosurgery provides the precise delivery of a single large dose of radiation to a target that typically measures less than 3.5 cm in diameter. This therapy has been used to treat tumors of the base of the skull and nasopharynx (Chou et al.).

Intraoperative Radiation Therapy

Intraoperative radiation therapy (IORT) provides a single large dose of electron beam radiation to a tumor bed during surgery. IORT is not used frequently but has been investigated for use in head and neck cancers (Chou et al., 2001).

Neutron and Proton Radiotherapy

Neutron and proton (particle) beam radiotherapies are under investigation for use in the treatment of head and neck cancers.

Brachytherapy

Brachytherapy is the temporary or permanent placement of a radioactive source either on or within a tumor. Brachytherapy also is called internal radiation or implant therapy. This therapy offers the advantage of delivering a high dose of radiation to a specific tumor volume with a rapid falloff in dose to adjacent normal tissues (Dunne-Daly, 1997). Brachytherapy can be classified as low dose rate (4–20 Gy/hr), medium dose rate (20–120 Gy/hr), or high dose rate (doses greater than 120 Gy/hr) (Boelsen & Jamar, 2000).

Brachytherapy can be performed on unresectable as well as resectable tumor areas of the head and neck. The radiation oncologist and head and neck surgeon work together in the operating room to place the brachytherapy catheters directly into the tumor. One or two days following surgery, the patient is taken to the radiation oncology department for loading of the catheters with iridium-192 radioactive seeds (Devine & Doyle, 2001). The treatment area then is x-rayed to verify the placement of the seeds. The patient returns to the inpatient room. The radiation oncologist and medical physicist determine the dosage and time needed to treat the cancer safely and adequately. After treatment is completed, the catheters and seeds are removed. An average brachytherapy treatment will range from 72–96 hours with an average dose of 30–40 Gy delivered. Brachytherapy also may be given in combination with EBRT. Brachytherapy techniques usually are temporary interstitial or intracavitary implants, but permanent interstitial implants also have been used for treatment of tumor extending into the base of the skull (Dunne-Daly, 1997).

Radiation Therapy Process

Consultation

A primary care provider, medical oncologist, or surgeon usually refers a patient with head and neck cancer to a radiation facility. The radiation oncologist performs an in-depth history and physical examination and evaluates previous staging studies (i.e., computed tomography [CT], magnetic resonance imaging, positron emission tomography scans). Surgical pathology is reviewed and staging is completed unless further studies are needed. The patient is counseled regarding the goals of RT as well as expected acute and chronic treatment side effects. If the patient consents to have treatment, the physician explains the consent forms and the patient signs them.

When the parotid gland is included in the radiation field, loss of saliva causes a dry mouth, or xerostomia, and results in the development of dental caries following treatment. Dental care and oral health are essential components of the treatment planning process. Therefore, patients with head and neck cancer must have a pretreatment prophylactic dental evaluation. Dental work, such as extractions, fillings, or gum surgery, must be done prior to RT. Patients are instructed in the use of custom-made fluoride trays molded for daily dental prophylaxis.

Prior to starting RT, patients having concurrent chemotherapy often will have a venous access device placed to allow adequate IV access for continuous chemotherapy. Most patients receiving RT to the head and neck also will require gastrostomy tube (GT) placement for alternative nutritional support because of acute dysphagia. Ideally, the GT should be placed prior to starting treatment to allow the insertion site time to heal so that the patient may lie flat during treatment without discomfort.

Simulation: Treatment Planning

Simulation is the planning process that allows the radiation oncologist to simulate a patient's treatment prior to starting therapy. Radiation treatments are planned by simulation with the use of fluoroscopy, x-ray films, or CT scanning to determine the target volume and parameters for treatment delivery. Simulation usually takes one to two hours. During this time, the patient is positioned lying on an x-ray table with an immobilization device in place (Holland, 2002). The immobilization device may be a soft, plastic mesh mask that is placed over the patient's face and molded to adhere closely. The patient can see and breathe normally through holes in the plastic mask. Some patients may experience increased anxiety related to the immobilization mask and may require medication prior to simulation. A custom-made bite block may be placed in the patient's mouth to maintain head position. The patient's shoulders also may be immobilized and pulled away from the treatment field by the use of handles similar to jump rope handles. These handles connect to a board at the patient's feet. Pressure from the patient's feet helps to hold tension on the ropes, thus pulling the shoulders down and out of the field. Tracheal and oral suctioning should be done before immobilization and during simulation as needed.

Tattoos are placed under the skin by pinpricks with black ink to permanently mark the radiation field. Tattoos also may be placed on the neck and supraclavicular region. To avoid placing tattoos on the patient's face, marks are made directly on the mask using a permanent marker to note treatment areas.

Templates of blocking, defining the treatment fields and shielding of normal structures, are drawn on the simulation x-ray planning films. With CT simulation, the physician can outline the tumor and normal structures on each CT slice. Following simulation, the medical physicist and dosimetrist determine an optimal dose distribution, and various field plans are generated for the radiation oncologist to review and approve (Holland, 2002). At this time, the physician will decide on the fractionation schedule, dose of treatment, and type of treatment (IMRT, 3DCRT, or traditional treatment fields) to be delivered.

Treatment

RT is delivered using a team approach. Each member of the treatment team performs an important role in a patient's care. See Figure 7-1 for members of the RT team.

Prior to starting RT, the patient must have treatment verification films taken and approved by the radiation oncologist. This process verifies the treatment fields and blocks. Often, minor improvements are made to the treatment plan at this

---

Figure 7-1. Radiation Therapy Team

- Radiation oncologist
- Radiation oncology nurse
- Medical physicist
- Dosimetrist
- Radiation technologist/therapist
- Medical secretaries
- Treatment assistant staff

---

time, and the process can take 30–60 minutes. The first treatment may be given once verification has been completed. Daily treatment times range from 10–20 minutes, depending on the number of treatment fields. Patients will undergo treatment Monday through Friday, five days a week, until the prescribed dose is reached. Port verification films are taken weekly for quality assurance to document the accuracy of the radiation treatment. The radiation oncologist sees patients once a week and as necessary for assessment and evaluation of side effects. Patients also consult with the radiation oncology nurse as problems arise during therapy.

Follow-Up Care

When the prescribed radiation treatments have been completed, patients undergo follow-up care. The radiation oncologist determines the frequency of follow-up visits. These visits may be as often as weekly or may be extended to months between visits. The surgeon and/or medical oncologist also routinely see patients for follow-up. It is during follow-up care that patients are monitored for resolution of acute side effects and surveillance of chronic side effects.

Side Effects

Major side effects of RT often are divided into three groups: acute, subacute, and chronic. Acute side effects occur during treatment or up to two weeks after treatment. They occur in most rapidly dividing cells, such as mucosal surfaces, gastrointestinal cells, hair follicles, bone marrow, and urinary bladder. Edema and inflammation in the normal tissues cause these side effects. Subacute side effects occur within three weeks to three months after treatment is completed. These side effects occur in more slowly dividing cells of the liver, bone, and endocrine tissues. Chronic side effects occur between four months and two years after RT. Chronic side effects occur in the most slowly dividing cells of the nerve, cartilage, and muscle tissue. Figure 7-2 lists specific side effects of RT to the head and neck area, which vary according to treatment fields. Each of these side effects will be reviewed at length along with the appropriate nursing care and patient education needed to care for a patient receiving RT to the head and neck.

Patient Education

The Oncology Nursing Society's (ONS) *Standards of Oncology Education: Patient/Significant Other and Public* stated that "education is a component of comprehensive nursing care for the patient and significant others experiencing cancer as well as the public" (Blecher, 2004, p. 2). Patient education is designed to effect changes in knowledge, attitudes, and behavior to promote coping (Clarke, 2002). Patients need

Figure 7-2. Side Effects of Treatment

Acute Side Effects
- Mucositis, oral infection, oral pain
- Dysphagia, odynophagia
- Esophagitis, pharyngitis
- Taste alterations, nutritional changes
- Xerostomia, secretion changes
- Nasal dryness
- Fatigue, depression
- Pain

Chronic Side Effects
- Laryngeal edema
- Radiation dermatitis, alopecia
- Dental caries, osteoradionecrosis
- Tissue fibrosis
- Ocular, otologic changes
- Thyroid dysfunction
- Spinal cord injury
- Xerostomia

information about their treatment, general emotional support, and practical help with side effects of treatment. To reduce anxiety and enhance self-care, the information should include the presentation, prevalence, and duration of side effects (Wengstrom & Forsberg, 1999).

Patients receiving RT require ongoing education throughout the course of treatment. Signs and symptoms as well as duration and management of treatment side effects must be discussed. The nurse, radiation oncologist, or radiation therapist may initiate teaching. Multidisciplinary patient and family education is an important aspect of patient care because RT is a frightening concept for the general public to grasp. Most information regarding radiation is felt to be negative. Turning these feelings into a positive experience is a challenge for the RT team. Teaching may be performed in a group setting or one-on-one using a variety of resources, such as verbal information, written information, video, or demonstration. Patient pathways are useful for educating patients with head and neck cancer regarding the RT experience. A patient pathway is a written patient education tool that maps or charts the expected course of treatment from the pretreatment phase through the recovery phase (Clarke, 2002).

Communication for patients with head and neck cancer often is impaired by tumor invasion or anatomical changes resulting from surgery. Patients may be in the early stages of speech therapy and unable to speak clearly; therefore, patience and consideration need to be implemented in these situations. Staff should encourage patients to write their questions and concerns and provide adequate time for this to occur.

Family members often are useful as interpreters for patients with impaired communication. Patients and families must be assessed for their level of understanding of the teaching delivered. Reinforcement of teaching must be offered throughout therapy.

Symptom Management

RT to the head and neck results in both acute and chronic side-effects. Nursing interventions are aimed at symptom management and patient education. In 1990, the ONS Radiation Therapy Special Interest Group established a work group to improve and standardize the documentation of nursing care provided to patients receiving RT. Improved documentation of side effect management and patient education also was a goal of this work group. As a result, ONS published the *Radiation Therapy Patient Care Record* (Catlin-Huth, Pollock, & Haas, 2002), which has become the standard RT documentation tool in healthcare facilities across the United States.

Mucositis, Oral Infection, and Oral Pain

Mucositis is defined as inflammation of the mucous membrane. Stomatitis refers specifically to inflammation of the oral cavity. Refer to Figure 7-3 for the National Cancer Institute's (2003) mucositis toxicity criteria.

Mucositis typically occurs during the first two weeks of RT because of the impaired ability of the epithelial cells to replicate and replenish (Gosselin & Pavilonis, 2002). More than 50 published papers in the nursing literature have documented the clinical investigations aimed at the prevention, palliation, or reduction of RT-induced oral mucositis in patients with head and neck cancer. The most effective measure to treat RT-induced mucositis is frequent oral rinsing with a bland mouthwash, such as saline or sodium bicarbonate rinse, to reduce the amount of microbial flora (Shih, Miaskowski, Dodd, Stotts, & MacPhail, 2002). Patients with severe stomatitis should not use hydrogen peroxide rinses because new tissue is easily broken down by hydrogen peroxide.

Infection of the oral mucosa often is seen in patients receiving head and neck RT. Oral infections may be caused by bacteria (e.g., *Pseudomonas, Klebsiella, Staphylococcus, Streptococcus*) or fungus (e.g., *Candida*). Culture and sensitivity studies are necessary to treat bacterial infections appropriately. Fungal infections usually present as a burning sensation of the tongue and mucous membranes and the appearance of small white patches ("cottage cheese") in the oral cavity. Antifungal therapy may be necessary throughout RT.

Figure 7-3. Grading of Mucositis Caused by Radiation

0—None
1—Erythema of the mucosa
2—Patchy pseudomembranous reaction (patches generally ≤ 1.5 cm in diameter and noncontiguous)
3—Confluent pseudomembranous reaction (contiguous patches generally > 1.5 cm in diameter)
4—Necrosis or deep ulceration; may include bleeding not induced by minor trauma or abrasion

Note. Based on information from National Cancer Institute, 2003.

Oral pain from mucositis or oral infection must be treated promptly and effectively. Topical oral rinses may coat or numb areas of discomfort temporarily. Nonsteroidal anti-inflammatory drugs and/or narcotics may be indicated for moderate to severe pain. Liquid or transdermal routes of administration may be a better alternative to pills for patients with head and neck cancer. See Figure 7-4 for nursing interventions useful for the patient with mucositis.

Figure 7-4. Nursing Interventions for Mucositis

- Encourage frequent mouth care, q 2–4 hours, especially after meals and at bedtime.
- Provide frequent mouth rinses with salt water and/or sodium bicarbonate solution.
- Recommend avoiding commercial mouth care products and lemon/glycerine swabs.
- Recommend avoiding irritating substances such as cigarettes, alcohol, and spicy or acidic foods.
- Recommend a soft toothbrush or foam swabs for oral care.
- Instruct the patient to remove dentures between meals and at bedtime.
- Treat dentures with antifungal prescription medication if a fungal infection is present.
- Encourage the completion of antifungal or antibiotic therapy as prescribed.
- Recommend eating foods that are cold or room temperature; hot foods may be more irritating.
- Encourage the use of topical/systemic measures prescribed to ease pain.
- Assess the patient's pain level as often as necessary to maintain comfort.
- Assess oral mucosa weekly and as needed for infection.
- Educate the patient to perform oral inspection daily and to report changes immediately.

Dysphagia, Odynophagia, and Esophagitis

Dysphagia is defined as the inability to swallow or difficulty swallowing; odynophagia is painful swallowing; and esophagitis is inflammation of the esophagus. These acute side effects may occur when a patient is receiving radiation to the throat and upper chest, usually starting within two weeks of treatment and subsiding two or more weeks after treatment is completed. Figure 7-5 lists the most appropriate nursing interventions.

Taste Alterations and Nutritional Changes

Dysgeusia is the perversion of the gustatory sense where normal tastes are interpreted as unpleasant or different from the characteristic taste of a particular food or chemical compound.

Ageusia is the absence, partial loss, or impairment of the sense of taste. Prolonged alteration in taste sensation is an anticipated and unpleasant side effect of head and neck radiation. Taste alterations may appear subtle and become more pronounced as treatment continues. Taste alteration may take

---

Figure 7-5. Nursing Interventions for Dysphagia, Odynophagia, and Esophagitis

- Suggest that patient consume soft, moist foods that have minimal irritation to the esophagus.
- Avoid hot or cold extremes in temperature; room temperature foods may be more soothing.
- Provide straws for drinks and a cup or glass instead of a bowl and spoon for soups.
- Encourage topical/systemic pain medication prior to meals.
- Weigh the patient at least once a week.

---

up to six or more months to return to normal. Some patients report permanent taste alteration.

Nutritional changes occur for multiple reasons, such as taste alteration, anorexia, mucositis, and fatigue. It is important to educate the patient and family on the importance of good nutrition during RT. See Figure 7-6 for nutritional nursing interventions.

Xerostomia and Secretion Changes

Xerostomia is dryness of the mouth caused by a reduction in the amount of saliva produced. Xerostomia occurs when the salivary glands (parotid, submandibular, and sublingual) receive significant exposure in the radiation treatment field. Patients may experience xerostomia during the first week of treatment, and it is thought to be permanent once the RT exceeds 40–50 Gy (Brizel et al., 2000). Xerostomia is both an acute and chronic side effect of RT. Acutely, the saliva becomes thick, ropey, and tenacious. Salivary fibrosis leads to the chronic state of xerostomia. Xerostomia may result in tenderness, burning and/or pain in the oral cavity, difficulty wearing dentures, and difficulty eating, speaking, and sleeping. These side effects significantly impact a patient's quality

---

Figure 7-6. Nursing Interventions for Improved Nutrition

- Encourage small, frequent meals (five to six per day).
- Choose and prepare foods that look and smell good.
- Marinate meat, chicken, or fish with mild seasoning or sweet fruit juice.
- Use bacon, ham, or onion to flavor bland foods.
- Instruct the patient to rinse his or her mouth with baking soda solution prior to meals to moisten mucosa and stimulate taste buds.
- Recommend high-calorie liquids or nutritional supplements.
- Instruct the patient on ways to increase the calorie content of food.
- Suggest eating foods at room temperature, which may be more palatable.
- Recommend the use of plastic utensils and plates to decrease metallic taste.
- Encourage the patient to eat with others or while watching TV.
- Weigh the patient frequently.
- Consult with a dietitian as needed.

of life (Gosselin & Pavilonis, 2002). Figure 7-7 lists nursing interventions for patients with xerostomia.

Two medications have been developed to reduce the chronic side effect of radiation-induced xerostomia. Oral pilocarpine (Salagen®, MGI Pharma, Bloomington, MN) is a salivary stimulant that can be used during and after RT. If effective, pilocarpine can be taken daily for the patient's lifetime. Pilocarpine tablets are prescribed at an initial dose of 5 mg three times a day, and the dose can be adjusted according to therapeutic response, up to 30 mg per day. The most common side effect is sweating. Chills, flushing, headache, and frequent urination also may occur.

Amifostine (Ethyol®, MedImmune, Gaithersburg, MD) is a cytoprotectant that selectively protects normal tissues from the effects of chemotherapy and/or radiation. Amifostine accumulates in many epithelial tissues, with the highest concentrations found in the salivary glands and kidneys (Brizel et al., 2000). The U.S. Food and Drug Administration has approved amifostine for use in patients who are undergoing postoperative radiation for head and neck cancer when the radiation port includes a substantial portion of the parotid gland (Gosselin & Pavilonis, 2002). Although amifostine generally is well tolerated, nausea, vomiting, and hypotension are the most commonly reported side effects (Brizel et al.). Antiemetics and prehydration are essential for patients to tolerate amifostine treatment. Amifostine is given daily prior to RT.

Figure 7-7. Nursing Interventions for Xerostomia

- Confirm that a dental evaluation has been done prior to therapy.
- Encourage the patient to follow the mouth care regimen provided by his or her dentist.
- Suggest the patient moisten his or her mouth frequently with water, artificial saliva, or sugar-free liquids.
- Suggest frequent oral rinses with salt water and/or sodium bicarbonate solution.
- Suggest the use of a humidifier to decrease mucosal dryness.
- Order home suction equipment as needed.
- Increase the patient's intake of fluids to at least 8–10 glasses a day.
- Encourage the use of Biotène® (Laclede, Rancho Dominguez, CA) mouth care products.
- Suggest foods with sauces, gravies, and salad dressing to make them moist and easier to swallow.
- Encourage the use of lip balm to relieve lip dryness.
- Suggest the use of sugar-free candy or gum to moisten mouth.

Nasal Dryness

Cancers of the sinus and nasopharynx may require the administration of RT to the nasal passages. The nasal mucosa may become very dry and irritated, leading to cracking and

bleeding. Mucous secretions become dry, hard, and crusty, making them hard to remove with nose blowing. See Figure 7-8 for nursing interventions for nasal dryness.

Figure 7-8. Nursing Interventions for Nasal Dryness

- Encourage a fluid intake of 8–10 glasses throughout the day.
- Suggest the use of a humidifier, especially at night in the bedroom.
- Administer saline nasal spray to moisten nasal passages.
- Apply petroleum or hydrocortisone ointment intranasally to moisten the membrane and provide comfort.
- Consult with the otorhinolaryngology department for nasal lavage for obstructive secretions.

Laryngeal Edema

Laryngeal edema is swelling of the larynx and can be caused by RT. Symptoms of edema of the larynx include hoarseness, dyspnea, and stridor, which require intubation or tracheostomy. Voice changes usually will progress during radiation and improve slowly after therapy is completed. Figure 7-9 lists nursing interventions for laryngeal edema.

Figure 7-9. Nursing Interventions for Laryngeal Edema

- Assess the patient's voice quality weekly.
- Monitor for symptoms of breathing difficulty (stridor/dyspnea).
- Encourage frequent gargling with salt water and/or sodium bicarbonate solution.
- Encourage the patient to rest voice.
- Explain voice quality changes to the patient and family.
- Administer steroids, as ordered, to decrease swelling.

Radiation Dermatitis and Alopecia

Radiation dermatitis is an expected side effect of RT. Most patients receiving RT to the head and neck will have some degree of skin reaction as a result of normal tissue breakdown from ionizing radiation. Skin reactions may include mild to brisk erythema, dry or moist desquamation, or skin necrosis and ulceration of the dermis (NCI, 2003). Nursing interventions for dermatitis are listed in Figure 7-10.

Moist desquamation results from the inability of the basal layer to proliferate sufficiently to replace the epidermal surface (Sitton, 1998). Moist desquamation may be painful for the patient. Like many radiation side effects, skin reaction usually will begin two to three weeks after the start of treatment and continue for two to four weeks after treatment is completed.

Alopecia is hair loss caused by follicular death because of RT. For the patient with head and neck cancer, alopecia results in loss of facial hair in addition to the loss of scalp

---

Figure 7-10. Nursing Interventions for Dermatitis

- Teach the patient and family proper skin care during radiation therapy, including
  - Use mild soap.
  - Avoid friction when washing and rinse completely with water.
  - Use an electric razor for shaving.
  - Avoid the use of shaving creams or aftershave lotion.
  - Avoid the use of perfume and make-up.
  - Avoid sun exposure to treatment areas; wear a hat and clothing to protect skin.
  - Moisturize skin three times a day with recommended gels or creams.
  - Use hydrocortisone cream for itchy skin.
  - Do not apply skin care products for two to four hours before the radiation treatment, depending on product used.
  - Avoid tight-fitting clothing that may cause irritation of the treatment area.
- For the patient with moist desquamation,
  - Avoid gauze dressings that stick and may cause bleeding.
  - Do not apply tape to skin in the radiation treatment area.
  - Nonstick dressings may be useful.
  - Antibiotic ointment combined with lidocaine may comfort the reaction area.
  - Give pain medication as prescribed.

---

hair, depending on the treatment field. Hair growth usually will return six to eight weeks after RT, but the growth may be patchy and thin. Patients must be prepared for the cosmetic changes that may appear.

Skin care products used to treat radiation dermatitis vary among institutions. Nurses should be aware that some patients might be predisposed to skin problems. Nurses must be aware of newly developed products and research regarding these products so that effective treatment can be instituted. Recent research done by Olsen et al. (2001) demonstrated that adding aloe vera gel to a patient's skin care regimen may offer a protective effect. Aloe vera gel is low cost and usually easy to find, unlike many other skin care products.

Dental Caries and Osteoradionecrosis

Patients receiving ionizing radiation to the parotid glands usually develop xerostomia. Even with recent advances in medication, it is not really known if saliva after RT has the same chemical composition as prior to RT. Saliva is composed of electrolytes and minerals, small organic molecules and essential proteins that continually coat the oral mucosa. Patients with xerostomia are at increased risk for dental decay (dental caries) because of the inability of saliva to lubricate and cleanse the mouth and act as a buffer to acid.

Osteoradionecrosis/chondronecrosis is radiation injury to the bone or cartilage. Irradiation can adversely affect cellular elements of bone, which can limit the potential for wound maintenance and ability to heal after a traumatic event. Elective oral surgical procedures are contraindicated within an irradiated field. If surgical intervention (e.g., extractions,

endodontic or periodontal surgery) is required after RT, pre- and postoperative hyperbaric oxygen treatments may increase the potential for healing and minimize the risk for osteoradionecrosis. See Figure 7-11 for nursing interventions.

Tissue Fibrosis and Trismus

Soft tissue fibrosis is the development of firmness of the soft tissues of the neck. Trismus is the tightening of the mastication muscles in the jaw, which, if not prevented or treated, can significantly hinder the patient's ability to chew. Nursing interventions include

- Encourage frequent exercises such as chewing exercises.
- Refer patient to physical therapy for a dynamic bite opener.
- Make dietary changes as needed.
- Assess the mouth opening measurement periodically.

Ocular and Otologic Changes

Radiation can cause injury to the structures of the eyes. Careful planning is performed to avoid treating these structures whenever possible. If the area surrounding the eye must be treated, a lead shield may be placed under the eyelid to block the radiation from injuring the eye.

Serous otitis media is the development of sterile fluid within the middle ear. In some situations, patients have drainage tubes surgically placed in the ear. Earwax can become hard within the ear canal, and an ear, nose, and throat specialist must lavage and remove the hard wax. Nurses should assess patients for hearing changes.

Hypothyroidism

Hypothyroidism is the decreased function of the thyroid gland. This is a subacute side effect of RT. Thyroid-stimulating hormone levels should be monitored and Synthroid® (Abbott Laboratories, North Chicago, IL) prescribed to treat this problem. Once patients are diagnosed with hypothyroidism, they will need to take Synthroid for life, and dose adjustments will be made often. Hypothyroidism left untreated can cause weight problems, fatigue, and hair changes.

Spinal Cord Injury

Radiation-induced myelopathy is injury to the spinal cord that could result in paralysis. Lhermitte sign is characterized by shock-like sensations that radiate down the back and

---

Figure 7-11. Nursing Interventions for Dental Care

- Confirm that the patient has had a prophylactic dental evaluation.
- Encourage compliance with prescribed treatments, such as
  - Fluoride applications daily for life.
  - Regular brushing and flossing.
  - Avoiding candy, gum, and drinks high in sugar.
  - Rinsing often.

---

extremities when the neck is flexed. Often, these symptoms pass with time; sometimes a neck collar is prescribed to help with discomfort. Fortunately, with today's knowledge of radiobiology and availability of sophisticated treatment planning techniques, radiation injury to the spinal cord is avoidable in most situations (Hilderley, 1997).

Fatigue and Depression

Most patients receiving head and neck radiation experience fatigue to some degree. The actual mechanism of fatigue has not been clearly defined but appears to be related to the presence of excess toxic metabolites and waste products of cell destruction (Hilderley, 1997). Nutrition, sleep patterns, mucosal discomfort, secretion management, and daily activity all can impact fatigue.

Depression often is seen in patients with head and neck cancer. Rose and Yates (2001) reported a moderate level of perceived depression in patients receiving RT for cancers of the head and neck. Patients need monitoring and professional intervention for depression. Figure 7-12 lists nursing interventions for fatigue and depression.

Figure 7-12. Nursing Interventions for Fatigue and Depression

- Teach the patient to reduce activity levels when tired.
- Encourage frequent naps or rest periods throughout the day.
- Limit the patient's naps to one to two hours so that the patient can sleep at night.
- Increase the patient's hours of sleep at night with earlier bedtimes or sleeping in.
- Encourage the use of sleep medication as prescribed.
- Recommend short periods of light exercise to decrease fatigue.
- Encourage the use of pain medication as prescribed so the patient may be more comfortable at sleep times.
- Encourage the patient to maintain high-calorie/high-protein intake to improve energy level.
- Refer the patient to a social worker for emotional, spiritual, and financial support as needed.

Summary

RT is an important treatment modality in the management of head and neck cancer. Recent advances in technology have dramatically changed the delivery of RT to the head and neck area. Patients with head and neck cancer require complex patient management guided by a dedicated healthcare team. Nursing care has become highly specialized within the realm of radiation oncology nursing practice. In particular, the role of the nurse is inherent in providing the patient and family with the information necessary to understand the anticipated treatment course and to adequately manage treatment side effects.

References

Al-Sarraf, M. (2002). Treatment of locally advanced head and neck cancer: Historical and critical review. *Cancer Control, 9,* 387–399.

Ang, K., Peters, L., Weber, R., Morrison, W., Frankenthaler, R., Garden, A.S., et al. (1994). Postoperative radiotherapy for cutaneous melanoma of the head and neck region. *International Journal of Radiation Oncology, Biology, Physics, 30,* 795–798.

Berkowitz, D., & Malin, M. (2002). The revolution in radiation therapy. *Journal of Oncology Management, 11*(1), 15–24.

Blecher, C.S. (Ed.). (2004). *Standards of oncology education: Patient/significant other and public* (3rd ed.). Pittsburgh, PA: Oncology Nursing Society.

Boelsen, R., & Jamar, S. (2000). Advances in radiation oncology. *Oncology Nursing Updates: Patient Treatment and Support, 7*(3), 1–11.

Brizel, D., Wasserman, T., Henke, M., Strnad, V., Rudat, V., Monnier, A., et al. (2000). Phase III randomized trial of amifostine as a radioprotector in head and neck cancer. *Journal of Clinical Oncology, 18,* 3339–3345.

Catlin-Huth, C., Pollock, V., & Haas, M. (Eds.). (2002). *Radiation therapy patient care record: A tool for documenting nursing care.* Pittsburgh, PA: Oncology Nursing Society.

Chou, R., Wilder, R., Wong, M., & Forster, K. (2001). Recent advances in radiotherapy for head and neck cancers. *ENT—Ear, Nose, and Throat Journal, 80,* 704–719.

Clarke, L.K. (2002). Pathways for head and neck surgery: A patient-education tool. *Clinical Journal of Oncology Nursing, 6,* 78–82.

Devine, P., & Doyle, T. (2001). Brachytherapy for head and neck cancer: A case study. *Clinical Journal of Oncology Nursing, 5,* 55–57.

Dunne-Daly, C. (1997). Principles of brachytherapy. In K.H. Dow, J.D. Bucholtz, R. Iwamoto, V. Fieler, & L.J. Hilderley (Eds.), *Nursing care in radiation oncology* (2nd ed., pp. 21–35). Philadelphia: W.B. Saunders.

Gosselin, T.K., & Pavilonis, H. (2002). Head and neck cancer: Managing xerostomia and other treatment induced side effects. *ORL—Head and Neck Nursing, 20*(4), 15–21.

Hilderley, L.J. (1997). Principles of teletherapy. In K.H. Dow, J.D. Bucholtz, R. Iwamoto, V. Fieler, & L.J. Hilderley (Eds.), *Nursing care in radiation oncology* (2nd ed., pp. 6–20). Philadelphia: W.B. Saunders.

Hoffman, H.T., Karnell, L.H., Funk, G.F., Robinson, R.A., & Menck, H.R. (1998). The National Cancer Data Base Report on cancer of the head and neck. *Archives of Otolaryngology—Head and Neck Surgery, 124,* 951–962.

Holland, J. (2002). External beam radiation therapy. *ADVANCE for Nurses, 6*(7), 17–19.

National Cancer Institute. (2003). *Common terminology criteria for adverse events* (Version 3.0). Bethesda, MD: Author. Retrieved January 20, 2005, from http://ctep.cancer.gov/reporting/ctc.html

Olsen, D.L., Raub, W., Bradley, C., Johnson, M., Macias, J.L., Love, V., et al. (2001). The effect of aloe vera gel/mild soap versus mild soap alone in preventing skin reactions in patients undergoing radiation therapy. *Oncology Nursing Forum, 28,* 543–547.

Rose, P., & Yates, P. (2001). Quality of life experienced by patients receiving radiation treatment for cancers of the head and neck. *Cancer Nursing, 24,* 255–263.

Rose-Ped, A.M., Bellm, L.A., Epstein, J.B., Trotti, A., Gwede, C., & Fuchs, H.J. (2002). Complications of radiation therapy for head and neck cancers: The patient's perspective. *Cancer Nursing, 25,* 461–467.

Shih, A., Miaskowski, C., Dodd, M.J., Stotts, N.A., & MacPhail, L. (2002). A research review of the current treatments for radiation-induced oral mucositis in patients with head and neck cancer. *Oncology Nursing Forum, 29,* 1063–1080.

Sitton, E.L. (1998). Nursing implications of radiation therapy. In J.K. Itano & K.N. Taoka (Eds.), *Core curriculum for oncology nursing* (3rd ed., pp. 616–629). Philadelphia: W.B. Saunders.

Wengstrom, Y., & Forsberg, C. (1999). Justifying radiation oncology nursing practice. A literature review. *Oncology Nursing Forum, 26,* 741–750.

CHAPTER 8

Chemotherapy

Jill Solan, RN, MS, ANP, OCN®, and
Mary Jo Dropkin, PhD, RN

Introduction

Chemotherapy first was used to treat head and neck cancer in the early 1960s and, along with radiation therapy (RT), remains standard treatment to control local disease by overcoming radioresistance and addressing microscopic disease (Al-Sarraf, 2002). In the mid-1970s, chemotherapy use expanded to treat unresectable stage IV head and neck cancer, and it continues to play a major role in treating unresectable and/or metastatic disease. The focus on combining chemotherapy agents to enhance effectiveness began in the 1980s. Cisplatin plus 5-fluorouracil was and still is the most commonly used chemotherapy combination for treating head and neck cancer.

Following the success of a number of clinical trials using chemoradiation regimens for treating cancers of the larynx, nasopharynx, and oropharynx, the use of chemotherapy as initial therapy has increased. Several successful treatment regimens emerged in the 1980s. Clinical trials aimed at larynx preservation led to the use of chemotherapy as the standard treatment for stage III and IV resectable cancers of the larynx. RT for nasopharynx cancer allowed high locoregional and metastatic disease rates to persist, but by adding the radiosensitizing chemotherapy agents cisplatin and 5-fluorouracil to the RT regimen, five-year survival has improved (Al-Sarraf, 2002). Novel biologic targeted therapies hold promise but need further investigation to determine whether these agents are effective in treating head and neck cancer.

Principles of Treatment

Neoadjuvant therapy refers to the use of chemotherapy alone as initial treatment or chemotherapy administered prior to standard therapy. *Adjuvant* chemotherapy follows standard therapy to augment the potential success of surgery or RT in patients at high risk for recurrence. Chemotherapeutic agents usually are combined with RT to treat cancers of the head and neck because chemotherapy alone has proved to be ineffective in treating advanced epithelial cancers in which cure is the goal. Prior to starting any treatment regimen, however, tumor factors, host factors, and drug factors must be considered (Pfister, 2003) (see Figure 8-1).

Tumor factors include histology, or cell type, grade, tumor volume, vascularity of the tumor, and previous treatment, such as surgery or RT. Medical comorbidity, performance status, compliance, immune status, and extent of prior treatment all are host factors that are taken into consideration. Finally, drug factors, such as type and dose of agent, single agent or combination therapy, route of administration, combination

---

Figure 8-1. Factors to Consider Before Beginning Treatment

Tumor Factors
- Histology
- Grade
- Tumor volume
- Vascularity of the tumor
- Previous treatment

Host Factors
- Medical comorbidity
- Performance status
- Compliance
- Immune status
- Extent of prior treatment

Drug Factors
- Type and dose of agent
- Single agent versus combination therapy
- Route of administration
- Combination with definitive locoregional therapy
- Timing of administration: sequential versus concomitant
- Therapeutic index: toxicity and side effects

Note. Based on information from Pfister, 2003.

---

with definitive locoregional therapy, timing of administration (sequential versus concomitant), and the therapeutic index, or toxicity and side effects, are critical in making decisions regarding the treatment regimen (Pfister, 2003).

Sequential Versus Concomitant Chemotherapy

In general, the administration of chemotherapy is based on the principles of pharmacokinetics, including absorption, distribution, metabolism, and excretion (Tortorice, 1997). Subsequently, the goal of treatment and the biochemical nature of the agent are critical factors in determining the chronology of administration. Sequential chemotherapy occurs when a preselected number of chemotherapy cycles is administered and the response is evaluated before deciding to proceed with another form of treatment. Concomitant, or concurrent, chemotherapy occurs when chemotherapy cycles are administered according to a specific protocol at the same time RT is being administered (Pfister, 2003). Several randomized trials have demonstrated that an integrated chemotherapy/RT program improves control rates relative to those obtained by RT alone with unresectable squamous cell carcinoma of the head and neck (Al-Sarraf et al., 1998; Brizel et al., 1998; Weissler et al., 1992; Wendt et al., 1998). Similar results occurred in patients with advanced oropharynx cancers and nasopharynx cancer (Calais et al., 1999). These results are particularly important for patients with nasopharynx cancer because of its propensity for distant metastases (Al-Sarraf et al.).

A number of approaches to concomitant chemoradiotherapy are available, such as single-agent chemotherapy, combination chemotherapy with split-course RT, and alternating chemotherapy with RT. Within these schemes, the treatment can be altered. The treatment variables that commonly are altered include the chemotherapy agent and dose; the timing of administration of the chemotherapy; and the dose, fraction size, and fractionation schedule of RT (Pfister, 2003). The tumor's response to chemotherapy can indicate that the tumor is radiosensitive; thus, the combination of chemotherapy and RT can have a synergistic effect.

The use of combination chemotherapeutic agents has proved to be more effective than single-agent therapy but may be associated with a higher degree of toxicity. Furthermore, concomitant regimens can cause side effects and toxicities that have a severe impact on the patient's quality of life (Rose-Ped et al., 2002). Often, these problems are acute and manageable, but some sequelae of treatment are chronic and require both physical and psychological adaptation by the patient.

In summary, the clinical evidence to date has shown that concomitant chemoradiotherapy is the current treatment of choice for many head and neck cancers. Chemotherapy acts as a radiosensitizer, improving cure rates but possibly exacerbating the side effects of RT. Finally, the combined use of chemotherapeutic agents may increase the risk of side effects and toxicities versus a single-agent chemotherapy regimen.

In this case, split-course radiation, in which RT and chemotherapy are administered alternately, allows patients to recover from each treatment's side effects (Harris, 2000).

Organ Preservation

Traditionally, the treatment for most advanced, resectable epithelial cancers of the head and neck was surgery with postoperative RT. Chemotherapy was considered for recurrent, unresectable, or metastatic disease. The goal for these patients was palliative control, not cure of the disease. Throughout the past decade, however, chemotherapy has become a major part of a multimodality regimen to treat advanced cancers of the upper aerodigestive region (larynx, nasopharynx, oropharynx), with the focus on preservation of organs and structures that are essential for speech and swallowing (Maluf, Sherman, & Pfister, 2001). A number of randomized trials have evaluated concurrent chemotherapy and RT versus RT alone for the purpose of organ preservation (Weber et al., 2003).

Beginning in the 1980s, the Department of Veterans Affairs Laryngeal Cancer Study Group (1991) launched the first trial of induction chemotherapy plus RT. After the cycles of neoadjuvant chemotherapy (two to three cycles given every three weeks) were completed, the tumor response was evaluated, and the patients received RT. This trial laid the groundwork for other regimens to be studied for larynx preservation and for treatment of cancers of the hypopharynx (Department of Veterans Affairs Laryngeal Cancer Study Group). More recently, researchers have determined that combined modality treatment (chemotherapy/RT) with surgery (reserved for salvage) significantly improves larynx preservation in patients with advanced cancers of the larynx and hypopharynx (Maluf et al., 2001).

Cancers of the oropharynx, which include tumors of the base of the tongue and tonsil, are other examples of head and neck primary sites that have been treated successfully with chemoradiotherapy regimens designed for organ preservation (Pfister, 2003). Concomitant regimens use both standard and hyperfractionated RT. The goal of a nonsurgical approach with cancer of the oropharynx is to maintain the functions of swallowing and speech.

Ongoing Clinical Research

In general, studies are ongoing to determine which chemotherapeutic agents are effective in treating squamous cell carcinoma of the head and neck and which treatments will result in an immediate and sustained cure for primary locoregional control and prevention of distant metastasis. Specifically, research is needed to determine which chemotherapeutic agents are most effective in improving cure rates and controlling locoregional disease and distant metastasis (Aliff, West, & Pfister, 2002). Side effects of chemoradiotherapy are significant, and some treatment sequelae persist throughout the patient's life. Additional quality-of-life studies are needed to investigate whether function is, in fact, maintained by organ preservation and whether this will have a positive impact on the quality of life of the patient with head and neck cancer (Rose-Ped et al., 2002).

Patients with early cancers or premalignant lesions receive chemopreventive agents to reduce the risk of future cancers. Some of the agents studied include a class of oral vitamin A analogs called retinoids and COX-2 inhibitors. Retinoids can reduce precancerous lesions, but when discontinued, the lesion can regrow. Ongoing placebo-controlled randomized trials are being pursued and are an area of great interest (Aliff et al., 2002).

The Nursing Role

The nurse holds multiple responsibilities in chemotherapy treatment. The administration of chemotherapy requires specialized nursing education and supervised training that follow guidelines established by the Oncology Nursing Society to ensure that adequate hydration, premedication, antiemetics, and chemotherapy are administered properly (Polovich, White, & Kelleher, 2005). Chemotherapy doses are based on the patient's body surface area and are calculated based on the patient's height and weight. The oncology nurse must be knowledgeable about the drug to be delivered, including the dosage, route of administration, and the overall sequelae that can occur. The nurse also must be familiar with venous access devices and infusion pumps and follow Occupational Safety and Health Administration guidelines for safe handling of cytotoxic agents (Polovich, 2003). Oncology nurses provide education to patients and caregivers regarding the prevention and management of treatment side effects. A thorough health history and physical assessment must be an ongoing process, beginning with pretreatment and continuing during treatment and post-treatment. Any change in health history, including pain and difficulty breathing, swallowing, or talking, must be noted and communicated to the healthcare team. As the patient proceeds through treatment, a focal assessment of the head and neck region, particularly the oral cavity, is critical. A thorough oral examination at each patient encounter must include the condition of the lips, gums, teeth, oral mucosa, tongue, tonsils, and uvula. This examination is critical in evaluating the patient's tolerance of treatment, determining if the patient is becoming nutritionally compromised or dehydrated, and identifying the need for any revisions to the nursing plan of care (Weber & Kelley, 2003). Xerostomia (Maher, 2004) and mucositis (Beck, 2004) are particularly common in patients undergoing chemotherapy and RT and significantly can decrease quality of life, depending on level of morbidity. Examination of the nose and sinuses is similarly important in those patients being treated for cancer of the nasopharynx.

Fatigue is the most commonly reported side effect of cancer treatment and can occur during or after chemotherapy. The nurse should discuss energy conservation techniques with the patient, including resting prior to activity and ensuring adequate hydration and nutrition with an emphasis on consuming a high-protein/high-calorie diet (Gosselin & Pavilonis, 2002; Nail, 2004).

Because nausea and vomiting can occur soon after the administration of chemotherapy, it is essential that patients take antiemetics as prescribed. Caregivers should measure urine output and maintain the patient's hydration.

Finally, these patients are at significant risk for infection. It is important to monitor them carefully for neutropenia, altered skin integrity, altered mucosal barrier (Wujcik, 2004), and anemia (Nail, 2004).

Summary: Nursing Role

Treatment of head and neck cancer can be emotionally challenging for both the patient and caregiver. Nursing assessments should include patient coping strategies. Referrals for psychological counseling and/or support group participation should be considered. If the patient demonstrates a prolonged inability to cope, then a psychiatric referral is warranted for evaluation and treatment of depression or other maladaptations.

Additional nursing responsibilities include active communication with patients, physicians, and other members of the treatment team if the patient is experiencing any signs of adverse reaction, side effects, or toxicities from chemotherapy; administration of hydration, premedication, antiemetics, and the chemotherapy agent according to protocol; education of patients and caregivers on prevention and management of treatment side effects, particularly focusing on what adverse reactions may occur and to whom adverse reactions should be reported; and provision of ongoing emotional support.

Chemotherapeutic Agents Used to Treat Head and Neck Cancers

The chemotherapy agents used to treat head and neck cancers are cisplatin, carboplatin, 5-fluorouracil, paclitaxel, doxorubicin, methotrexate, and bleomycin. The following section describes each of these agents in detail.

Cisplatin

Cisplatin (also known as cisplatinum, Platinol® [Bristol-Myers Squibb, Princeton, NJ], and CDD) does not induce oral mucositis or increase the local toxicity of RT in head and neck cancer. It is the best radiosensitizer (Al-Sarraf, 2002).
Classification: Alkylating agent
Route: IV

Mechanism of action: Breaks the DNA helix strand, thereby interfering with DNA replication.

Side effects:
- Severe nephrotoxicity
- Nausea and vomiting
- Myelosuppression
- Ototoxicity: sensorineural hearing loss and tinnitus
- Neurotoxicity
- Hyperuremia
- Hypersensitivity reaction
- Hypomagnesemia
- Peripheral neuropathy

Nursing considerations and management:
- Cisplatin has a vesicant potential if > 20 cc 0.5 mg/ml is extravasated. In lower doses, cisplatin is an irritant (Dorr, 1994).
- The drug should be held if serum creatinine is > 1.5 mg/dl to prevent irreversible renal tubular damage.
  - Amifostine may be used as a renal protectant because it selectively protects normal tissue from the effects of chemotherapy and RT (Gosselin & Pavilonis, 2002).
  - Amifostine is broken down by alkaline phosphatase in the tissue to the active metabolite thiol. This active metabolite is found in normal tissues and detoxifies the reactive metabolites of cisplatin (Spratto & Woods, 2004).
  - Amifostine also has been used to prevent and minimize xerostomia, which is significant in patients receiving RT for head and neck cancer (Brizel et al., 2000).
- Vigorous hydration is needed to prevent nephrotoxicity. Mannitol is administered to achieve osmotic diuresis.
- A baseline audiogram should be obtained because the drug is potentially ototoxic (Polovich et al., 2005).

Patient education:
- Immediate side effects (within 24 hours)
  - Nausea or vomiting can begin within 2 hours after receiving cisplatin and can last for 24 hours. Nausea may continue or recur for several days.
  - Loss of appetite may occur 24–48 hours after treatment.
  - Allergic reactions can occur but are rare.
- Early side effects (within one week)
  - Diarrhea may occur but usually subsides within a day.
  - Kidney damage may occur unless cisplatin is given with large amounts of IV and oral fluids. Hydration is essential before, during, and after treatment.
  - A ringing (tinnitus) or "stuffed" sensation in the ears or difficulty hearing may occur within one week after treatment and may persist. The "stuffed" sensation usually subsides in two to three weeks.
- Late side effects (after one week post-treatment)
  - A temporary decrease in red and white blood cell and platelet counts. This may occur 7–14 days after treatment. This usually is mild and does not warrant any

intervention or alteration in dosage or treatment plan.
  - Temporary thinning or loss of hair may occur several weeks after treatment.
  - Numbness, tingling, or burning in the hands and feet may occur after several treatments but are uncommon.
- Additional information to provide to the patient
  - Cisplatin may cause temporary or permanent effects to hearing, such as ringing or stuffed sensation in the ears, loss of high-frequency hearing, and difficulty hearing in background noise.
  - Cisplatin may be damaging to the kidneys; therefore, hydration and adequate fluid intake are required.
  - Antiemetics should be taken as instructed (see Table 8-1). Doses should not be skipped even if no nausea is noted.
  - Aspirin, ibuprofen, and similar products should NOT be taken.
  - The physician or nurse should be advised if the patient is taking any over-the-counter preparations (e.g., herbal supplements) because some can interfere with the actions of chemotherapy.

Carboplatin

Carboplatin (also known as Paraplatin® [Bristol-Myers Squibb]) has an action similar to cisplatin, but with different side effects (Al-Sarraf, 2002).

Classification: Alkylating agent

Route: IV

Mechanism of action: Breaks the DNA helix strand, thereby interfering with DNA replication.

Side effects:
- Thrombocytopenia
- Neutropenia (Myelosuppression is more pronounced with renal impairment.)
- Nausea and vomiting
- Renal and hepatic toxicity (uncommon)

Nursing considerations and management: (Polovich et al., 2005)
- Carboplatin exhibits less toxicity than cisplatin; therefore, rigorous hydration usually is not necessary.
- Monitor blood counts closely and reduce doses per protocol.
- If needed, administer prescribed growth factors to treat myelosuppression (neutropenia, anemia).
- Monitor for fever of 100.5°F (38.0°C) or higher.

Patient education:
- Early side effects (Cleri & Haywood, 2002)
  - Although rare, an allergic reaction, such as flushing, shortness of breath, low blood pressure, skin rash, or erythema, can occur during administration of carboplatin. Anaphylactic-like and allergic reactions can occur within minutes of beginning administration of the drug.

Table 8-1. Antiemetic Agents

Agent	Indications	Mechanism of Action	Recommended Dosing	Nursing Considerations
Serotonin receptor antagonists: ondansetron, granisetron, dolasetron	Acute nausea related to moderately to highly emetogenic chemotherapy	Selectively block the stimulation of serotonin release and the effects of serotonin, both centrally (in the chemoreceptor trigger zone [CTZ] and vomiting center) and peripherally (in the gastrointestinal [GI] tract)	**Ondansetron hydrochloride (HCl):** 8 mg po 30 minutes before chemotherapy, then 4 and 8 hours after chemotherapy; then 8 mg po three times a day for 1–2 days; or 32 mg IV 30 minutes before chemotherapy; or three 0.15 mg/kg infusions 30 minutes before chemotherapy, with the second and third doses given 4 and 8 hours after the first dose; with highly emetogenic chemotherapy, administer 24 mg po 30 minutes before chemotherapy. **Granisetron HCl:** 10 mcg/kg via IV (over 5 minutes) 30 minutes before chemotherapy; or 1 mg po twice a day given 1 hour before chemotherapy, then 12 hours later; or 2 mg po every day 1 hour before chemotherapy **Dolasetron mesylate:** 100 mg po 1 hour before chemotherapy; or 1.8 mg/kg via IV 30 minutes before chemotherapy; or 100 mg via IV (over 30 seconds) 30 minutes before chemotherapy	Side effects include headache, diarrhea, and hypotension. Occasionally, dolasetron and ondansetron may cause acute, usually reversible, echocardiogram changes.
Corticosteroids: dexamethasone, methylprednisolone	In combination with serotonin receptor antagonists for acute and delayed emesis associated with moderately to highly emetogenic chemotherapy; OR in combination with a substituted benzamide or phenothiazine for moderately emetogenic chemotherapy; OR alone in patients receiving moderately emetogenic chemotherapy	Unclear; may be because of the release of endorphins or to prostaglandin antagonism	**Dexamethasone:** 20 mg via IV or po before chemotherapy for prevention of acute nausea and vomiting; for delayed nausea and vomiting, 8 mg twice a day for 2–3 days, then 4 mg twice a day for 1–2 days, then discontinue **Methylprednisolone:** 40–125 mg IV before chemotherapy	Usually is contraindicated in patients receiving biotherapy Dose should be tapered if used for more than several days. Careful monitoring is required in patients with diabetes mellitus. Dexamethasone is the corticosteroid most often used for control of delayed nausea and vomiting. Side effects include anxiety, insomnia, acne, and appetite changes. Long-term use may result in Cushingoid syndrome, psychosis, seizure, and other adverse effects.

(Continued on next page)

Table 8-1. Antiemetic Agents (Continued)

Agent	Indications	Mechanism of Action	Recommended Dosing	Nursing Considerations
Substituted benzamides: metoclopramide	Alone OR in combination with a corticosteroid for control of acute nausea and vomiting caused by moderately emetogenic chemotherapy; OR alone for delayed nausea and vomiting	At lower doses, antagonizes the dopamine receptors in the CTZ and the GI tract; at higher doses, also acts as a serotonin receptor antagonist	**Metoclopramide:** 10–20 mg po or 2–3 mg/kg via IV before chemotherapy and 2 hours after chemotherapy	Associated with a high incidence of extrapyramidal effects, especially in younger patients; should be given with diphenhydramine to minimize these effects IV administration is associated with significant cardiovascular side effects, including hypotension, bradycardia, and tachycardia. Side effects include dystonia, akathisia, diarrhea, sedation, and dry mouth.
Phenothiazines: prochlorperazine, perphenazine	Acute nausea and vomiting associated with moderately emetogenic chemotherapy; OR in combination with a corticosteroid for delayed nausea and vomiting; OR in combination with other agents in persistent nausea and vomiting	Acts primarily in the CTZ as a dopamine 2 receptor antagonist; also decreases vagal nerve stimulation of the vomiting center	**Prochlorperazine:** 10–20 mg po every 3–4 hours; 15–30 mg extended-release spansule po every 12 hours; 25 mg PR every 4–6 hours; 10–30 mg via IV every 3–4 hours **Perphenazine:** 1–5 mg via IV every 4–6 hours; may be given as a continuous IV infusion at a rate not greater than 1 mg/minute; 4 mg po every 4–6 hours; maximum of 15 mg per 24 hours (outpatient) or 30 mg per 24 hours (inpatient)	Associated with a high risk of extrapyramidal symptoms, especially in younger patients; may be given with diphenhydramine to minimize these effects Side effects include dystonia, sedation, photosensitivity, orthostatic hypotension, and akathisia
Butyrophenones: droperidol, haloperidol	Acute and delayed nausea and vomiting associated with moderately emetogenic chemotherapy	Blocks dopamine 2 receptors in the CTZ and vomiting center; also decreases stimulation of the vomiting center via the vestibular pathway.	**Droperidol:** 2.5–10 mg via IV every 3–4 hours; 0.5–2.5 mg via IV every 3–4 hours **Haloperidol:** 2–5 mg po every 4 hours; 0.5–2 mg via IV or IM every 2–6 hours	Associated with extrapyramidal symptoms, especially in younger patients; may be given with diphenhydramine to minimize these effects Use with caution in patients with cardiac disorders. Side effects include dystonia, akathisia, sedation, tachycardia, and hypotension.
Cannabinoids: dronabinol	Moderately emetogenic chemotherapy. Not a first-line antiemetic medication	Unclear; the active ingredient in cannabis may inhibit prostaglandin synthesis or indirectly block the vomiting center.	**Dronabinol:** 2.5–10 mg po two or three times a day	Can produce physical and psychological dependency Side effects include mood changes; drowsiness; impaired perception, sensory function, and coordination; tachycardia; hypotension; and appetite stimulation.

(Continued on next page)

		Table 8-1. Antiemetic Agents *(Continued)*		
Agent	**Indications**	**Mechanism of Action**	**Recommended Dosing**	**Nursing Considerations**
Benzodiazepines: alprazolam, lorazepam	Anticipatory nausea and vomiting; in addition to other agents to treat persistent nausea and vomiting. Not a true antiemetic, but may be useful as an adjunct to antiemetic medications	Antiemetic activity unclear; reduces anxiety by potentiating the activity of gamma-amino butyric acid in the brain	**Alprazolam:** 0.25–0.5 mg po two or three times a day **Lorazepam:** 1–3 mg po or sublingually every 4–6 hours; 0.5–2.5 mg IV or IM every 4–6 hours	Side effects include sedation, dizziness, and orthostatic hypotension.

Note. All doses listed are for adults. Based on information from American Society of Health-System Pharmacists, 1999; Gralla et al., 1998; Polovich et al., 2005; Skidmore-Roth, 2002; Spratto & Woods, 2002. From "Antiemetic Therapy in Patients Receiving Cancer Chemotherapy," by C. Marek, *Oncology Nursing Forum, 30,* pp. 263–264. Copyright 2003 by the Oncology Nursing Society. Adapted with permission.

- Diarrhea can occur the day of treatment but usually subsides within 24 hours.
- Mild nausea and vomiting occur within 24–72 hours after receiving the drug and can last for a few days.
• Late side effects (Cleri & Haywood, 2002)
- A decrease in white blood cells, red blood cells, and platelets can occur 7–21 days after treatment.
- Numbness, tingling, and burning in the hands or feet can occur after several treatments and is more common in patients older than 65 years of age. Overall, this reaction is uncommon.
• Additional information to provide to the patient
- This medication may cause temporary or permanent effects to hearing, such as ringing or a stuffed sensation in the ear, loss of high-frequency hearing, and difficulty hearing in background noise. This is more common in patients who are receiving aminoglycosides.
- The physician or nurse should be advised if the patient is taking any prescribed or nonprescribed medication when receiving carboplatin.
- Aspirin, ibuprofen, or any aspirin-containing products should not be taken unless prescribed by the doctor.
- Increase fluid intake for one week following treatment.
- Be aware of a decrease in urination.
- Excessive nausea, vomiting, or diarrhea and an inability to eat or drink for more than 24 hours after receiving carboplatin may require hydration/intervention.
- Observe for signs of bleeding, such as dark or tarry stool, bruising, faint red rash, and infection.

Fluorouracil

Also known as 5-FU and Adrucil® (SICOR Pharmaceuticals, Irvine, CA), this antineoplastic antimetabolite is used in conjunction with other chemotherapeutic agents in treating squamous cell carcinoma of the head and neck. It is administered intravenously and widely distributed throughout the body, including the central nervous system. It may be associated with neutropenia and oral or gastrointestinal ulceration (Lehne, 2004).

Classification: Antimetabolite

Route: IV

Mechanism of action: Acts in S phase and inhibits enzyme production for DNA synthesis, leading to strand breaks or premature chain termination.

Side effects: (Polovich et al., 2005)
• Myelosuppression
• Nausea
• Anorexia
• Vomiting
• Diarrhea
• Mucositis
• Alopecia
• Photosensitivity
• Darkening of the veins
• Dry skin
• Cardiac toxicity (rare)

Nursing considerations and management: (Cleri & Haywood, 2002; Polovich et al., 2005)
• Sun exposure increases skin reactions. Educate the patient about photosensitivity precautions to be followed; patient should wear protective clothing and sunscreen when in the sun.
• Leucovorin is given after chemotherapy to rescue normal cells from adverse reactions (Polovich et al., 2005; Spratto & Woods, 2004).

Patient education:
• Early side effects
- Mild nausea and vomiting
- Diarrhea
- Mucositis
• Late side effects (Cleri & Haywood, 2002)
- Temporary decrease in white blood cell and platelet counts may occur one to two weeks after treatment.

- Darkening of the nail beds, the skin, and the veins in which the drug was given may begin four to six weeks after receiving the drug and may persist.
- Temporary thinning of the hair may occur three to four weeks after each treatment.
- Photophobia, conjunctivitis, and watering of the eyes may occur three to four weeks after treatment.
• Additional information to provide to the patient
- Avoid taking aspirin, ibuprofen, or any aspirin-containing products unless prescribed by the doctor.
- Protect the skin from exposure to the sun. Wear sunscreen with a sun protection factor (SPF) of 15 or greater and protective clothing when in the sun.
- Observe for
  * A fever of 100.5°F (38.0°C) or higher
  * More than three loose bowel movements a day over normal routine
  * Black bowel movements, bruising, faint red rash, or any other signs of bleeding
  * Mouth sores
  * Unexpected or unexplained problems
  * Any questions or concerns (Memorial Sloan-Kettering Cancer Center, 2002).

Paclitaxel

Paclitaxel, also known as Taxol® (Bristol-Myers Squibb), acts to inhibit cellular division. It is widely distributed throughout the body, except to the central nervous system. Neutropenia can be a significant dose-limiting consideration (Lehne, 2004).

Classification: Taxane
Route: IV
Mechanism of action: Stabilizes microtubules to inhibit cell division. Effective in G2 and M phases. Interferes with cancer cells' ability to grow.
Side effects: (Polovich et al., 2005)
• Myelosuppression
• Alopecia
• Peripheral neurotoxicity
• Hypersensitivity reaction
• Facial flushing
• Myalgia
• Fatigue
• Cardiac arrhythmia
Nursing considerations and management: (Cleri & Haywood, 2002; Polovich et al., 2005)
• Do not use in pediatric patients.
• Pretreat to prevent hypersensitivity reactions, including anaphylaxis.
- Cimetadine 300 mg IV 30–60 minutes before treatment (unless contraindicated)
- Diphenhydramine 50 mg IV 30–60 minutes before treatment (unless contraindicated)

- Dexamethasone 20 mg IV 30–60 minutes before treatment
- Follow specific institutional guidelines, if available.
• Filter paclitaxel with 0.2 micron in-line filter.
• Use glass bottles or non–polyvinyl chloride (PVC) (such as polyolefin or polypropylene) bags to administer paclitaxel. Do not give paclitaxel with PVC bags or PVC tubing.
• Paclitaxel is an irritant. Extravasation may lead to local pain, edema, and erythema at the infusion site, but not skin necrosis (Ignoffo, Viele, Damon, & Venook, 1998; Polovich et al., 2005).
Patient education:
• Early side effects
- Patients may develop an allergic reaction within the first 15–60 minutes of treatment. Symptoms include urticaria, facial flushing, or trouble breathing. Premedication should be administered to prevent an allergic reaction.
- Mild nausea and vomiting, although uncommon, may occur while taking paclitaxel.
- Fatigue can occur during treatment.
- Joint pain and body aches may occur and usually can be relieved with acetaminophen or ibuprofen.
• Late side effects
- Mucositis may develop after four to seven days.
- Temporary partial or complete alopecia may occur depending on treatment schedule.
- Numbness, tingling, and pain in hands and feet may occur.
- Neutropenia, thrombocytopenia, and anemia may occur 7–10 days after treatment.
• Additional information to provide to the patient
- Concomitant use of ketoconazole may result in decreased metabolism of the paclitaxel.
- Use reliable contraception during treatment and for four months after treatment has ended (Spratto & Woods, 2004).
- Observe for
  * Fever higher than 100.5°F (38.0°C)
  * Mucositis
  * Decreased intake of food and fluids
  * Joint and back aches and pain not relieved by acetaminophen or ibuprofen
  * Uncontrolled nausea or diarrhea.

Less commonly used antineoplastic agents used to treat head and neck cancer include doxorubicin, methotrexate, bleomycin, etoposide (VP16), and ifosfamide.

Doxorubicin

Doxorubicin (Adriamycin® [Bedford Laboratories, Bedford, OH]) is a vesicant that has a dose-limiting cardiotoxicity. Antitumor antibiotics, in general, originated from cultures of streptomyces. They are used only in the treatment of cancer, not infection. Use of doxorubicin is limited, primarily in relation to cardiotoxicity (Lehne, 2004).

Classification: Antitumor antibiotic

Route: IV

Mechanism of action: Binds with DNA, thereby inhibiting DNA and RNA synthesis. Often used in combination to treat anaplastic thyroid cancer.

Side effects: (Cleri & Haywood, 2002; Polovich et al., 2005)

- Myelosuppression
- Nausea
- Vomiting
- Alopecia
- Mucositis
- Dose-limiting cardiotoxicity
- Photosensitivity
- Radiation recall
- Drug may turn urine red.

Nursing considerations and management: (Polovich et al., 2005)

- Doxorubicin is a vesicant.
- Doxorubicin may cause flare reaction.
- Check patient's ejection fraction via multiple-gated acquisition (MUGA) scan prior to starting treatment.
- Do not exceed a lifetime dose of 550 mg/m^2 (450 mg/m^2 if patient has had prior chest irradiation or concomitant cyclophosphamide treatment).
- Initiate dexrazoxane for patients who have received a cumulative dose of 300 mg/m^2 and are continuing doxorubicin treatment.

Patient education:

- Immediate side effects (beginning within 24 hours)
  - Itching, hives, or a red rash can occur at the injection site and along the vein while the drug is being given. This subsides as soon as the injection of the drug is completed. Instruct the patient to tell the nurse if any pain is experienced at the IV site.
  - Extravasation can result in tissue necrosis. Careful assessment of the vein should be done before, during, and after administration of doxorubicin.
  - Nausea and vomiting can begin one to three hours after the drug is given and can last 24–48 hours.
  - Urine can be pink or red in color for as long as 48 hours after the treatment.
  - Palpitations
- Early side effects (beginning within one week)
  - Palpitations
  - Mucositis can develop.
- Late side effects
  - A temporary decrease in white blood cell and platelet counts can occur 10–14 days after each treatment.
  - Temporary thinning or loss of hair is common and can occur two to four weeks after each treatment.
  - Damage to the heart muscle can occur after a certain dose level is reached. MUGA scans, electrocardio-

grams, and echocardiograms are performed at periodic intervals to monitor the patient's status.
  - Redness of the skin can develop in an area where radiation has previously been given.
- Additional information to provide to the patient
  - Instruct the patient to take antiemetics as prescribed.
  - Instruct the patient to protect the skin from the sun by wearing sunscreen and protective clothing.
  - The patient should not take aspirin or ibuprofen unless prescribed.
  - Observe for
    * Fever
    * Signs of bleeding (dark, tarry stool, bruising of the skin)
    * Pain, burning, redness, swelling, or blistering near the injection site (Memorial Sloan-Kettering Cancer Center, 2002).

Methotrexate

Also known as MTX and Mexate® (Bristol-Myers Squibb), methotrexate is a folic acid analog that blocks the conversion of folic acid to its active form, thereby inhibiting cellular reproduction. Used with leucovorin rescue to enhance its effects (Lehne, 2004).

Classification: Antimetabolite

Route: IV

Mechanism of action: Acts in S phase; inhibits enzyme production for DNA synthesis, leading to strand breaks or premature chain termination. Used mainly for palliation in the patient with head and neck cancer.

Side effects: (Polovich et al., 2005)

- Mucositis
- Nausea
- Myelosuppression (especially as folic acid antagonist)
- Gastrointestinal ulceration
- Renal toxicity
- Photosensitivity
- Liver toxicity
- Neurotoxicity associated with high-dose MTX

Nursing considerations and management:

- Instruct the patient to avoid taking multivitamins with folic acid.
- Encourage good mouth care.
- Instruct the patient to protect the skin from the sun by wearing sunscreen with an SPF of 15 or greater and protective clothing (Polovich et al., 2005).

Bleomycin

Also known as Blenoxane® (Bristol-Myers Squibb), this agent binds to DNA, interfering with synthesis of DNA and, to a lesser extent, RNA and protein synthesis. Bleomycin has the potential to cause pulmonary toxicity (Spratto & Woods,

2004). Another antitumor antibiotic, bleomycin is unusual in that it is related to minimal bone marrow suppression. It can, however, cause severe long-term lung injury (Lehne, 2004).

Classification: Antitumor antibiotic

Route: IV, intramuscular, subcutaneous, or intrapleural

Mechanism of action: Binds with DNA, thereby inhibiting DNA and RNA synthesis.

Side effects: (Cleri & Haywood, 2002; Polovich et al., 2005)

- Hyperpigmentation
- Alopecia
- Photosensitivity
- Renal toxicity
- Hepatotoxicity
- Pulmonary fibrosis
- Fever
- Chills
- Hypersensitivity or anaphylactic reaction (rare)

Nursing considerations and management: (Cleri & Haywood, 2002; Polovich et al., 2005)

- Educate patient and family to disclose previous use of bleomycin if anesthesia is needed. Pulmonary toxicity may be enhanced with intraoperative forced inspiratory oxygen.
- Cumulative lifetime dose of bleomycin should not exceed 400 units. Higher doses can result in pulmonary fibrosis.

Issues Associated With Chemotherapy Treatment

Chemotherapy for head and neck cancer places both a physical and psychological demand on the patient and significant others. Many patients with cancer of the head and neck receive a combination of treatments, including surgery, chemotherapy, and RT.

Compliance is a major issue for patients, their families, and healthcare providers. Despite ongoing efforts, some patients do not access medical care when needed. A number of factors can influence compliance with treatment schedules and regimens. These include psychosocial factors, in which patients are lacking support from the family or community. Behavioral factors, such as alcohol abuse and addiction, may have caused the patient's lifestyle to exclude health care. Treatment requiring daily radiation and concomitant chemotherapy requires a commitment from both the patient and family. The patient often must rely on the family for transportation or other resources that may not be available. Compliance is a complex problem with many components that are unique to each patient and family.

Several nursing studies have described the difficulty patients experience in relation to treatment side effects from chemotherapy (Huang, Wilkie, Schubert, & Ting, 2000; Ohrn, Sjoden, Wahlin, & Elf, 2001) and chemoradiation (Rose-Ped

et al., 2002). But specific issues concerning symptom severity, compliance with treatment, and medical care access have not been empirically tested in this population from a nursing perspective. Nurses and all members of the healthcare team need to look at these issues to try to understand what barriers interfere with patients' compliance and what interventions may be effective in influencing compliance. Nurses are challenged to create innovative approaches and interventions that will facilitate patient compliance. When caring for this patient population, oncology nurses must be aware of the physical and psychological considerations involved with chemotherapy treatment.

Physical Considerations

Patients may have difficulty swallowing because of the disease and treatment. Also, sequelae of treatment often will make it impossible for patients to maintain nutrition by the oral route. Percutaneous endoscopic gastrostomy tube placement prior to treatment will ensure the patient receives adequate hydration and nutrition, including calories and protein. Patients need clear instruction regarding enteral therapy and medication administration.

To help to maintain oral hygiene, a humidifier can be used to provide supplemental moisture. This additional humidity is important for patients with xerostomia and dry skin. Oral irrigations with a mild salt or salt and baking soda solution and use of nonalcoholic mouth rinses should be routinely performed throughout the day, after meals, and at bedtime.

Because mucositis is a frequent side effect of chemotherapy, patients should be encouraged to use topical treatments to promote comfort, which should enable them to maintain nutrition. A mixture of equal parts of viscous lidocaine, diphenhydramine, and a liquid antacid provides temporary relief of pain, and the topical application of a suspension of sucralfate offers relief by providing a protective coating over damaged mucosa (Beck, 2004).

Assessment and treatment of pain related to both the cancer of the head and neck and the sequelae of treatment will be necessary. Commonly used medications for this patient population include fentanyl transdermal patches, codeine/oxycodone elixirs, and other drugs per institutional guidelines. Special care must be taken to begin a bowel regimen to prevent constipation depending on the chemotherapeutic agent and pain medication used.

Psychological Considerations

Listed as one of the most commonly experienced side effects related to therapies available to treat cancer, fatigue can be related to treatment or can result from disruption of sleep. The nurse should offer the patient and family resources as well as ways to minimize fatigue. Two Internet resources that offer suggestions for the management of cancer-related fatigue are the Oncology Nursing Society Fatigue Resource Area (http://onsopcontent.ons.org/Toolkits/Fatigue/index.shtml) and CancerSymptoms.org (http://cancersymptoms.org).

Another psychological consideration of cancer treatment is disruption in the patient's position and role in the family. Often, the patient undergoing treatment for cancer of the head and neck must rely on friends and family to help not only with activities of daily living but also with transportation and support.

Disruption of job/career also may result from cancer treatment. The patient with cancer of the head and neck may require prolonged treatment and have alterations in both appearance and function that may influence his or her ability to return to work. This can result in additional concerns about financial status and healthcare insurance.

Body image changes (e.g., tracheostomy, secretions) may affect the patient either temporarily or permanently. Body image is one's perception of his or her body, and many patients with cancer of the head and neck will require assistance in adapting to the changes. Depression and an altered quality of life may result from the body image change.

Patients may have concerns about the future in relation to the illness (e.g., "Am I going to survive, and if I'm cured, will my cancer come back?"). Survivorship issues are a concern of every patient with cancer, but the patient with head and neck cancer must adapt to not only the changes resulting from the treatment but also the poorer prognosis than that which may be seen with other tumor sites.

Summary

Although chemotherapy alone has not been effective in treating head and neck cancer, the combined use of chemotherapy and RT has proved to be successful in treating locally advanced squamous cell carcinoma of the head and neck. The combination of chemoradiation has allowed for organ preservation of the larynx and has led to ongoing clinical trials for squamous cell carcinoma of the oropharynx, tonsil, and base of the tongue to preserve functions such as speech and swallowing. Nasopharynx RT and chemotherapy are now the standard treatment for disease at this site.

Further prospective clinical trials are needed to find active chemotherapeutic agents that will have a sustained effect and benefit in controlling and curing cancer of the head and neck. New targeted therapies are using epidermal growth factor receptor (EGFR) blockers, EGFR monoclonal antibodies, and tyrosine kinase inhibitors aimed at blocking pathways that foster tumor growth. Further investigation in this area may hold future possibility to effectively treat head and neck cancers (Al-Sarraf, 2002).

Nurses continue to play a major role in educating the public about techniques to eliminate risk behaviors that cause head and neck cancer. Nurses are on the front lines in caring for patients and their caregivers throughout the course of treatment and recovery.

References

Aliff, T.B., West, A., & Pfister, D.G. (2002). Update: The role of chemotherapy in the treatment of squamous cell head and neck cancer. *News From SPOHNC (Support for People with Oral and Head and Neck Cancer), 12*(1), 1–6.

Al-Sarraf, M. (2002). Treatment of locally advanced head and neck cancer: Historical and critical review. *Cancer Control, 9,* 387–399.

Al-Sarraf, M., LeBlanc, M., Giri, P.G., Fu, K.K., Cooper, J., Vuong, T., et al. (1998). Chemoradiotherapy versus radiotherapy in patients with advanced nasopharyngeal cancer: Phase III randomized Intergroup Study 0099. *Journal of Clinical Oncology, 16,* 1310–1317.

American Society of Health-System Pharmacists. (1999). ASHP therapeutic guidelines on the pharmacologic management of nausea and vomiting in adult and pediatric patients receiving chemotherapy or radiation therapy or undergoing surgery. *American Journal of Health-System Pharmacists, 56,* 729–764.

Beck, S.L. (2004). Mucositis. In C.H. Yarbro, M.H. Frogge, & M. Goodman (Eds.), *Cancer symptom management* (3rd ed., pp. 276–287). Sudbury, MA: Jones and Bartlett.

Brizel, D.M., Albers, M.E., Fisher, S.R., Scher, R.L., Richtsmeier, W.J., Hars, V., et al. (1998). Hyperfractionated irradiation with or without chemotherapy for locally advanced head and neck cancer. *New England Journal of Medicine, 338,* 1798–1804.

Brizel, D.M., Wasserman, T.H., Henke, M., Strnad, V., Rudat, V., Monnier, A., et al. (2000). Phase III randomized trial of amifostine as a radioprotector in head and neck cancer. *Journal of Clinical Oncology, 18,* 3339–3345.

Calais, G., Alfonsi, M., Bardet, E., Sire, C., Germain, T., Bergerot, P., et al. (1999). Randomized trial of radiation therapy versus concomitant chemotherapy and radiation therapy for advanced-stage oropharynx carcinoma. *Journal of the National Cancer Institute, 91,* 2081–2086.

Cleri, L.B., & Haywood, R. (2002). *Oncology pocket guide to chemotherapy* (5th ed.). Philadelphia: Elsevier Science.

Department of Veterans Affairs Laryngeal Cancer Study Group. (1991). Induction chemotherapy plus radiation compared with surgery plus radiation in patients with advanced laryngeal cancer. *New England Journal of Medicine, 324,* 1685–1690.

Dorr, R.T. (1994). Pharmacologic management of vesicant chemotherapy extravasations. In R.T. Dorr & D.D. Von Hoff (Eds.), *Cancer chemotherapy handbook* (2nd ed., pp. 109–118). Norwalk, CT: Appleton & Lange.

Gosselin, T.K., & Pavilonis, H. (2002). Head and neck cancer: Managing xerostomia and other treatment induced side effects. *ORL—Head and Neck Nursing, 20*(4), 15–21.

Gralla, R.J., Navari, R.M., Hesketh, P.J., Popovic, W., Strupp, J., Noy, J., et al. (1998). Single-dose oral granisetron has equivalent antiemetic efficacy to intravenous ondansetron for highly emetogenic cisplatin-based chemotherapy. *Journal of Clinical Oncology, 16,* 1568–1573.

Harris, L.L. (2000). Head and neck malignancies. In C.H. Yarbro, M.H. Frogge, M. Goodman, & S.L. Groenwald (Eds.), *Cancer nursing: Principles and practice* (5th ed., pp. 1210–1243). Sudbury, MA: Jones and Bartlett.

Huang, H., Wilkie, D.J., Schubert, M.M., & Ting, L. (2000). Symptom profile of nasopharyngeal cancer patients during radiation therapy. *Cancer Practice, 8,* 274–281.

Ignoffo, R.J., Viele, C.S., Damon, L.E., & Venook, A. (1998). *Cancer chemotherapy pocket guide*. Philadelphia: Lippincott-Raven.

Lehne, R.A. (2004). *Pharmacology for nursing care* (5th ed.). St. Louis, MO: W.B. Saunders.

Maher, K. (2004). Xerostomia. In C.H. Yarbro, M.H. Frogge, & M. Goodman (Eds.), *Cancer symptom management* (3rd ed., pp. 215–229). Sudbury, MA: Jones and Bartlett.

Maluf, F.C., Sherman, E., & Pfister, D.G. (2001). Chemotherapy and chemoprevention in head and neck cancer. In J.P. Shah & S.G. Patel (Eds.), *Cancer of the head and neck* (pp. 444–461). Hamilton, Ontario, Canada: BC Decker.

Massaro, A.M., & Lenz, K.L. (2005). Aprepitant: A novel antiemetic for chemotherapy-induced nausea and vomiting. *Annals of Pharmacotherapy, 39,* 77–85.

Memorial Sloan-Kettering Cancer Center. (2002). *Patient information chemotherapy fact card.* New York: Author.

Nail, L.M. (2004). Fatigue. In C.H. Yarbro, M.H. Frogge, & M. Goodman (Eds.), *Cancer symptom management* (3rd ed., pp. 47–60). Sudbury, MA: Jones and Bartlett.

Ohrn, K.E., Sjoden, P.O., Wahlin, Y.B., & Elf, M. (2001). Oral health and quality of life among patients with head and neck cancer or haematological malignancies. *Supportive Care in Cancer, 9,* 528–538.

Pfister, D.G. (2003). Current status of chemotherapy. In J.P. Shah & S.G. Patel (Eds.), *Head and neck surgery and oncology* (3rd ed., pp. 663–672). Edinburgh, Scotland: Mosby.

Polovich, M. (Ed.). (2003). *Safe handling of hazardous drugs.* Pittsburgh, PA: Oncology Nursing Society.

Polovich, M., White, J.M., & Kelleher, L.O. (Eds.). (2005). *Chemotherapy and biotherapy guidelines and recommendations for practice* (2nd ed.). Pittsburgh, PA: Oncology Nursing Society.

Rose-Ped, A.M., Bellm, L.A., Epstein, J.B., Trotti, A., Gwede, C., & Fuchs, H. (2002). Complications of radiation therapy for head and neck cancers: The patient's perspective. *Cancer Nursing, 25,* 461–467.

Skidmore-Roth, L. (2002). *Nursing drug reference.* St. Louis, MO: Mosby.

Spratto, G., & Woods, A.L. (2004). *2004 edition PDR® nurse's drug handbook.* Clifton Park, NY: Thomson Delmar Learning.

Spratto, G.R., & Woods, A.L. (2002). *PDR nurse's drug handbook.* Montvale, NJ: Delmar.

Tortorice, P.V. (1997). Chemotherapy: Principles of therapy. In S.L. Groenwald, M.H. Frogge, M. Goodman, & C.H. Yarbro (Eds.), *Cancer nursing: Principles and practice* (4th ed., pp. 283–316). Sudbury, MA: Jones and Bartlett.

Weber, J., & Kelley, J. (2003). *Health assessment in nursing* (2nd ed.). Philadelphia: Lippincott Williams and Wilkins.

Weber, R.S., Berkey, B.A., Forastiere, A., Cooper, J., Maor, M., Goepfert, H., et al. (2003). Outcome of salvage total laryngectomy following organ preservation therapy: The Radiation Therapy Oncology Group trial 91-11. *Archives of Otolaryngology—Head and Neck Surgery, 129,* 44–49.

Weissler, M.C., Melin, S., Sailer, S.L., Qaqish, B.F., Roseman, J.G., & Pillsbury, H.C. (1992). Simultaneous chemoradiation in the treatment of advanced head and neck cancers. *Archives of Otolaryngology—Head and Neck Surgery, 118,* 806–810.

Wendt, T.G., Grabenbauer, G.G., Rodel, C.M., Thiel, H.J., Aydin, H., Rohloff, R., et al. (1998). Simultaneous radiochemotherapy versus radiotherapy alone for advanced head and neck cancer: A randomized multicenter study. *Journal of Clinical Oncology, 16,* 1318–1324.

Wujcik, D. (2004). Infection. In C.H. Yarbro, M.H. Frogge, & M. Goodman (Eds.), *Cancer symptom management* (3rd ed., pp. 252–275). Sudbury, MA: Jones and Bartlett.

CHAPTER 9

Postoperative Management of the Head and Neck Surgical Patient

Ann E.F. Sievers, RN, MA, CORLN

Introduction

Patients with head and neck cancer present postoperatively with multiple needs related to surgery that result in alterations in function and appearance. In addition, patients with head and neck cancer often present with comorbid conditions caused by the abuse of tobacco and alcohol, including peripheral vascular disease, liver disease, malnutrition, and chronic lung disease. In caring for these complex patients in the postoperative setting, nurses play an integral role as caregivers, teachers, advocates, counselors, and coordinators of care.

Multidisciplinary rounds representing each scientific discipline should be held on a regular basis to discuss patient care needs, team development, and team peer review. These meetings also provide for team support and bring synergy to the process. The treatment team includes staff nurses and clinical nurse specialists, physicians, nutritionists, oncology social workers, discharge planners, speech-language pathologists, physical therapists, occupational therapists, and psychiatrists. The oncology surgical nurse holds a unique and valued place as the treatment team's care coordinator because of the nursing focus on compassion, caring, and clinical competence (Krioukov, 1998).

Airway Management

Airway management is the main focus of nursing care for the patient undergoing surgery for head and neck cancer. Knowledge of the anatomy and physiology of the airway is key to competence and confidence in nursing management (see Figure 9-1). The nurse should be prepared to prevent problems and intervene in emergency situations in a calm and supportive manner.

Patients with head and neck cancer often present with a history of chronic obstructive pulmonary disease and chronic bronchitis resulting from a long history of smoking. Tidal volumes may be decreased with requirements for positive end expiratory pressure to maintain alveolar ventilation. Standard nursing care tasks, such as encouraging the patient to cough and deep breathe, are critical. An important and interesting aspect of head and neck surgery is that no interruption of the thorax or abdomen occurs during panendoscopy or surgical intervention; therefore, neither bellow dynamics nor the patient's lung capacity change. As a result, requirements for long postoperative ventilator time usually are limited.

It is not unusual for patients with head and neck cancer to present to a clinic or emergency room in airway distress or in extremis. The patient may be stridorous from a tumor

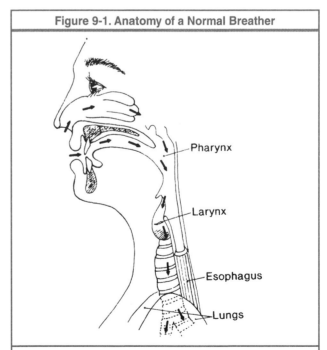

Figure 9-1. Anatomy of a Normal Breather

- Pharynx
- Larynx
- Esophagus
- Lungs

Note. From *Looking Forward: A Guidebook for the Laryngectomee* (3rd ed., p. 9), by R.L. Keith, 1995, New York: Thieme New York. Copyright 1995 by Thieme New York. Reprinted with permission.

obstructing the airway or from vocal cord paralysis. Nursing care should focus on positioning the patient at 45 degrees or higher to more properly align the airway and decrease dependent edema. IV access is necessary for medication administration, hydration, and steroid therapy. The patient should receive nothing by mouth (NPO) to prevent aspiration and prepare for possible tracheotomy. Interventions include the administration of nebulizer treatments, epinephrine, and slow IV hydration. Strict intake and output monitor fluid balance. Decreasing or limiting the patient's activity helps to conserve the work of breathing and promote oxygenation. Pulse oximetry is necessary to monitor oxygen saturation. Suction equipment must be available to effectively manage oral secretions. Obtain standard blood chemistry, hematocrit and hemoglobin, and arterial blood gases as ordered.

Because many chronically ill patients are anemic and have an impaired oxygen carrying capacity as well as chronic obstructive lung disease, they often require supplemental oxygen to maintain saturations above 95% (Pujade-Lauraine & Gascon, 2004). Limiting the patient's speaking and encouraging written communication will help to conserve energy. Place a tracheotomy tray or intubation tray at the bedside with appropriate sized airways. Pain medication, sedation, and anxiolytics should be administered judiciously to prevent further airway compromise.

Prepare the patient and family for the possibility of surgical intervention and the need for tracheotomy. If time permits, discuss with the patient and family the anatomic and functional changes that will occur following the procedure and alternate methods of communication. Although the capacity to learn during a crisis is limited, the conveyance of knowledge and engagement of trust between the nurse and the adult patient are crucial.

Nasal Obstructions

Similar interventions are appropriate for those patients with nasopharyngeal, nasomaxillary, and maxillary orbital tumors presenting with epistaxis and/or nasal obstruction. Using nasal packing to control nasal bleeding is the first intervention. Support of oxygenation and prevention of hypercarbia by monitoring arterial blood gases and pulse oximetry are nursing priorities. In most cases, these patients may not require surgical airway intervention. Multiple testing such as computed tomography (CT), magnetic resonance imaging, or CT angiography and embolization may be necessary. Nursing interventions center on airway maintenance, comfort, and the administration of pain medication.

Tracheotomy

A tracheotomy is a surgical incision into the trachea. The term "tracheostomy" refers to the actual opening into the trachea, or stoma (Tamburri, 2000). A tracheotomy often is performed in conjunction with intraoral, pharyngeal, hypopharyngeal, or laryngeal resections and neck dissections to avoid placement of an endotracheal tube in the surgical field and to prevent airway compromise caused by postoperative edema. In this situation, the tracheostomy usually is temporary but may remain in place for the duration of the postoperative course and, if required, through postoperative radiation therapy. A tracheostomy also can be permanent if airway compromise results from aspiration, surgically altered anatomy, or the need for postoperative chemotherapy and radiation therapy.

Tracheostomy Tubes

Tracheostomy tubes are selected based on specific patient needs (see Table 9-1). Tracheostomy tubes can be made of plastic (disposable) or stainless steel (reusable) and come in a variety of sizes, lengths, and diameters. The physician selects the size of the tube (length and diameter), which is determined by the patient's anatomy. Some tubes have only a single, outer cannula (no inner tube), whereas most tubes are double cannula with an outer cannula, an inner cannula, and an obturator (see Figure 9-2). The outer cannula remains in the patient at all times, except for routine changes. The inner cannula maintains a patent airway and is removed routinely for cleaning (Tamburri, 2000). The obturator is a stylet used for insertion of the entire tube and should remain with the patient at all times. A second tracheostomy tube of the same size and/or one size smaller should be available at the patient's bedside for immediate replacement in the event of inadvertent tube removal.

Tracheostomy tubes may be cuffed or uncuffed. A cuffed tube is placed during the surgical procedure and maintained until mechanical ventilation is no longer required and/or the patient is no longer at risk for aspiration. When inflated, the cuff seals the space between the tube and the trachea to provide a closed system for positive pressure ventilation, such as delivery of anesthesia or ventilator support (see Figure 9-3). The cuff is deflated when the patient is not on ventilator support or at risk for aspiration. The physician may write orders for cuff inflation indicating the reason for inflation, such as bleeding into the airway or documented aspiration. Patients who have undergone resection of sinonasal, nasomaxillary, or orbital carcinomas require cuff inflation for protection of dural repairs. This prevents pressure in the nasopharynx during peak ventilation and cough, allowing internal suture lines to heal without strain. When the cuff is inflated, cuff pressures should be checked every eight hours. Even high-volume, low-pressure cuffs can cause tracheal wall damage by impeding capillary blood flow to the tracheal mucosa. Cuff pressures should not exceed 20–25 mm Hg (Tamburri, 2000). An aneroid manometer placed on the cuff inflation valve measures cuff pressure.

The airway must be secure and in proper position. Circumferential tracheostomy ties are not indicated in the

Table 9-1. Tracheostomy Tubes

Type of Tracheostomy Tube	Description	Reason for Use
Cuffed	Standard tubes with low-pressure cuff and inner cannula, either reusable or disposable	Initial surgical tubes that are cuff inflated to create a sealed airway for artificial ventilation
Uncuffed	Standard tubes with no cuff; the inner cannula is either reusable or disposable; may be plastic or metal	Interim and permanent tubes used for airway access in the spontaneously breathing patient
Cuffed fenestrated	Standard tubes with cuff and fenestrated outer cannula; only in use when inner cannula is removed (unless inner cannula also is fenestrated)	Used almost exclusively for ventilator patients for speech when a cuff is required to seal the airway
Uncuffed fenestrated	Standard tube, no cuff, fenestrated outer cannula	May be used short term (one to three days) for weaning
Wire-reinforced silicone (also come in endotracheal lengths)	Wire-reinforced silicone covered tubes that, because of their internal integrity, will not lose their internal diameter in any position; some tubes have adjustable faceplates for exacting placement.	Operative tube; used when specific tip placement is required
Extra long	Tubes with longer shafts; usually made of more pliable material; standard tubes but can be custom made in lengths in the proximal or distal portion	Used in patients with excessive skin-to-trachea distance
Sleep apnea	Single-lumen tubes, pliable material; can be capped during the day and opened when asleep for sleep apnea	Used in patients with sleep apnea and patients with head and neck cancer who require slightly longer tubes, possibly because of reconstruction flaps around the airway
Laryngectomy	Shorter but with a larger relative inner diameter; crafted to the shape of a laryngectomy stoma with a more acute curve	After total laryngectomy, in cases where the stoma may be stenotic or obscured by reconstruction flaps or dressings
Laryngectomy buttons	Pliable material used with a pressure fit	For placement in the laryngectomy stoma to keep the airway patent; usually at the skin-trachea suture line
Custom-made	Any of the aforementioned tubes but with custom features to fit a particular patient; extra length, distal or proximal shape, cuff placement, short	Made-to-order tubes designed for a particular patient

presence of any type of reconstruction, flap, graft, or free flap. Rather, the ties should be suspended from secure points on each shoulder, so as not to put pressure over the reconstruction tissue. Velcro®-type ties or cotton tracheostomy ties secure the tracheostomy tube with the faceplate flush with the neck. The tube should be positioned in the center of the airway. If the tube is off center, determine the reason, ensure an adequate airway, and discuss the position with a physician.

Tracheostomy Care

Coughing and deep breathing, suctioning, and early ambulation are important aspects of care for the patient with an artificial airway. Tracheostomy care depends on the individual patient's needs and includes saline instillation, suctioning, coughing, surgical incision care, inner cannula care, and patient education directed at self-care. Postoperative head and neck surgery patients often have tenacious, bloody mucus and difficulty mobilizing secretions. The instillation of 3–5 cc of normal saline into the artificial airway every two to three hours will stimulate a cough and help to mobilize the secretions (Hudak & Bond-Domb, 1996). Encourage the patient to cough to clear secretions and determine the need for suctioning. Document the color, amount, and nature of secretions as well as the frequency of suctioning.

Remove and clean the inner cannula of the tube in a solution of equal parts of hydrogen peroxide and normal saline. If the inner cannula is disposable, replace it with a clean cannula matching the size of the tracheostomy tube. Clean the peristomal site at least every 8–12 hours with half-strength hydrogen peroxide, rinse with normal saline, and dry. Place a

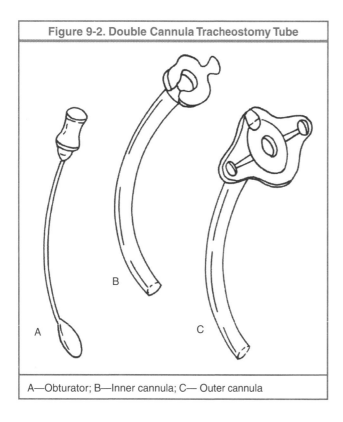

Figure 9-2. Double Cannula Tracheostomy Tube

A—Obturator; B—Inner cannula; C— Outer cannula

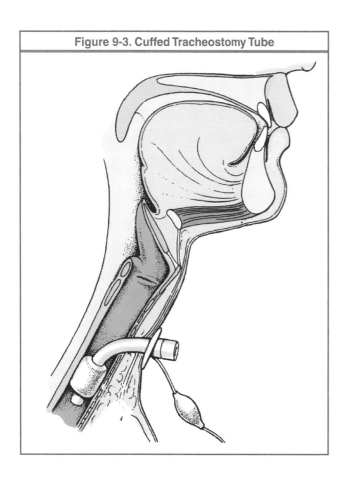

Figure 9-3. Cuffed Tracheostomy Tube

tracheostomy dressing under the faceplate of the tube to keep the site clean and dry. Cut gauze should not be used because the frayed fibers may be inhaled into the trachea or embedded in the wound (Tamburri, 2000). Placement of a skin protector, such as Stomahesive® (ConvaTec, Princeton, NJ), under the faceplate of the tube can prevent skin pressure erosion.

The normal upper airway mechanisms of warming, filtering, and moisturizing inspired air are bypassed when a tracheostomy is present. Supplemental humidity via a mist collar is necessary to protect the normal functioning of the mucociliary blanket and to prevent drying of the tracheal mucosa. Although controversial, strong clinical evidence has shown that saline instillation is very important to patients who are breathing unassisted through an artificial airway. A study by Hudak and Bond-Domb (1996) with postoperative head and neck surgery patients supported the use of saline following tracheotomy or laryngectomy to increase humidity and stimulate cough. The American Association of Critical-Care Nurses has published studies refuting saline instillation; however, these studies focus primarily on critical care patients who are on mechanical ventilators. This research should not be automatically applied to all patient populations (Raymond, 1995). Head and neck oncology nurses advocate the use of normal saline instillation and bedside home humidification (Hudak & Bond-Domb; Sievers & Donald, 1987).

Self-Care Teaching

If the patient is going home with a temporary or permanent tracheostomy, initiate self-care teaching early in the postoperative recovery period. This process begins by assessing the patient's readiness to learn. Determining whether the patient has seen himself or herself in the mirror is an important step as the patient begins to adapt to the physical changes related to the disease and surgical alterations (Clarke, 1998; Dropkin, 1989).

Make a contract with the patient for a time to begin teaching, and arrange for family members to be present. Demonstrate and explain each step of the procedure; assist the patient to return the demonstration. The nurse must supervise and observe the patient and family or significant other actually performing the procedures of airway care for 24–48 hours before hospital discharge. The goal is for the patient to demonstrate competence with saline instillation, wound care, suctioning, and inner cannula care. Discuss activities of daily living and emergency care and provide all instructions in writing. Make arrangements for the patient to have a suction machine and tracheostomy supplies at home and a homecare nurse for support and follow-up (Clarke, 1998).

Tracheostomy self-care teaching includes learning how to change the entire tracheostomy tube. The physician is responsible for the initial tracheostomy tube change, which usually occurs on the fifth postoperative day, when a well-defined tract has been formed (Hahn & Jones, 2000). Once the airway is stable, it is then safe for a nurse who is specially trained in this procedure to change the tube as ordered. Tube changes enhance hygiene, prevent scar stenosis, and minimize the formation of granulation tissue in the peristomal area. Many patients change the tube daily, but weekly changes usually are adequate. Ongoing evaluation of the patient's ability to safely perform his or her own care is integral to the education process and safe discharge.

Decannulation

Consider decannulation, or removal of a temporary trache-ostomy tube, when upper airway edema has subsided and the patient can swallow without evidence of aspiration. As with all procedures, the process should be explained to the patient to ensure understanding. Deflate the cuff of the tracheostomy tube and observe the patient's ability to manage secretions. Many physicians also will visually evaluate the integrity of the post-surgical airway by performing a fiberoptic endoscopy. Wean the patient from a temporary tracheostomy by downsizing the tube to a smaller, uncuffed tube to allow for air to flow around the tube into the natural larynx. The patient is taught to cover the tube with a finger when speaking or coughing. Place a cork, or decannulation stopper, in the outer cannula, allowing the patient to breathe through the nose and mouth and to speak (Tamburri, 2000). A tracheostomy speaking valve also can be placed on the inner cannula to permit the patient to speak. The return of speech is an acknowledged sign of progress. The patient must be able to coordinate breathing and exhalation with speaking to use either a valve or finger occlusion.

When preparing the patient for decannulation, the trache-ostomy tube is capped in the morning to allow for a full day of observation. Monitor oxygen saturation and airway comfort. Uncap the tube if the patient is having any airway distress to allow for unobstructed flow of air. Initially, the patient may be uncapped at night, but a trial of capping during sleep is indicated before removing the tube.

Remove the tracheostomy tube if the patient tolerates capping for 24 hours. Place the patient in a sitting position, and remove the tube in a downward and curved motion. Place an occlusive dry dressing over the incision and change it when soiled or wet. Instruct the patient to place two fingers over the dressing when talking or coughing to create a seal and promote wound healing. The incision should heal within three to five days. Document the patient's tolerance of the procedure in the chart.

Specialty Tracheostomy Tubes

Specialty tracheostomy tubes often are necessary because of alterations in anatomy, either natural or created by a surgical defect. Longer tubes may be required because of anatomic changes, obesity, the presence of reconstruction flaps, or increased skin-to-trachea distance. These usually are single cannula tubes with no inner cannula to remove and clean. Maintain the inner lumen with an increase in humidifica-tion using normal saline and mist. Suction the lumen of the tube because secretions often adhere to the distal tip of the tracheostomy tube.

Total Laryngectomy

A total laryngectomy is the removal of the larynx that results in a complete surgical disconnection between the airway and digestive tract. The trachea is sutured to the front of the neck, creating a permanent airway or stoma (see Figure 9-4). The upper airway (nose and mouth) no longer functions to warm, filter, or humidify air. The patient cannot speak with a normal voice but is able to eat without risk of aspiration. Nursing care focuses on airway and wound management and communication. The inner wall of the laryngectomy stoma should look similar to the oral mucosa—pink, moist, and glistening. During the healing process, the stoma may be compromised by edema, surgical reconstruction flaps, or the presence of sutures and may require placement of a laryngec-tomy tube or stoma button.

The nursing focus for the patient after a total laryngec-tomy is to maintain a patent airway. A flashlight or headlight should be at the bedside at all times because proper lighting is imperative to inspect the stoma for crusts and secretions. Bayonet forceps are useful in removing crusts.

When working with a patient with a stoma, the nurse should be protected from the patient's secretions by wearing safety

Figure 9-4. Anatomy of a Total Neck Breather (Laryngectomee)

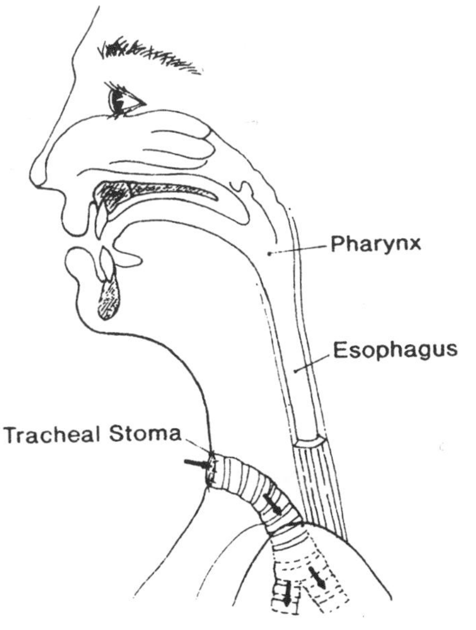

Pharynx

Esophagus

Tracheal Stoma

Note. From *Looking Forward: A Guidebook for the Laryngec-tomee* (3rd ed., p. 9), by R.L. Keith, 1995, New York: Thieme New York. Copyright 1995 by Thieme New York. Reprinted with permission.

eyeglasses and gloves. Stoma care will become easier once the sutures are removed.

Self-care teaching begins early in the postoperative period. The patient should begin to perform stoma and wound care as soon as possible. Instruct and support the patient in learning to cover the stoma, rather than the mouth, when coughing. Educate the patient and family regarding the effects of dry air on the airway. Using a small spray bottle, spray normal saline directly into the stoma. Small particle deposition is an excellent way to add moisture to the airway. At home, bedside humidifiers or cool mist vaporizers can provide additional moisture, particularly with low indoor humidity during the winter. Showers and steam rooms are very helpful for additional moisture. Change of seasons and the inability of the patient with a laryngectomy to quickly adapt to dryness may result in tracheitis and an occasional need for hospitalization. The use of a continuous ultrasonic nebulizer, systemic antibiotics, and triple antibiotic ointment applied to the stoma may prevent further crusting and infection.

Patients with an artificial airway or after total laryngectomy are unable to close their glottis to generate the pressure necessary to produce a normal cough or a Valsalva. This inability to Valsalva, in addition to the use of narcotic analgesics, can lead to constipation. A bowel regimen must become a routine part of life for these patients.

Airway Complications

Most airway complications can be prevented by addressing airway needs on a continuous basis (see Table 9-2). Surgical complications include subcutaneous emphysema, bleeding from a slipped ligature, and pneumothorax, as the upper lobes of the lung rise above the clavicle and sometimes into the surgical field.

Pain Management

Preoperative Pain

Alleviation of pain is a primary nursing function, and pain assessment is an ongoing process. Consider the location, severity, aggravating factors, and relieving factors. Pain management begins preoperatively when the patient presents with pain related to the tumor. Complaints may include sore throat, odynophagia, and unilateral otalgia. Aggressive pain management and patient and family education help to create a trusting relationship between the patient and nurse that will continue throughout the postoperative course.

Postoperative Pain

Following surgery, patients often describe relief from the pain that was caused by the tumor burden. The cause of postoperative discomfort is edema, numbness, and long immobility. Acute pain results from surgical incisions and tissue manipulation. However, the presence of multiple incisions and the use of flaps and grafts increase the number of potentially painful sites. Pain usually is short term, of moderate to severe intensity, and described as "sharp or burning." Pain also

Table 9-2. Preventable Airway Complications		
Type	**Signs and Symptoms**	**Nursing Care/Intervention**
Obstruction	• Speech without covering tube • "Snoring" with a tracheostomy • Unable to suction via the tube	Humidity, saline, suctioning, inner cannula care, changing the entire tube on a regular basis
Malposition	• Movement of the tube with respiration • Unable to suction via the tube • Patient talking without covering tube • Patient short of breath or uncomfortable	Apply faceplate to the skin, secure with ties or Velcro straps, and resecure often. Appropriate size tube for the trachea-to-skin distance Investigate the reason if unable to suction via the tube.
Bleeding	• Frank blood, crusting, clots • Pulsing of the tube	Airway humidification, saline Sign of possible innominate artery rupture
Air in neck	• Subcutaneous air	Decrease pressure if patient is on a ventilator.
Communication with wound	• Saliva via tracheostomy tube or tracheostomy wound	Impeccable wound care and packing
Pneumothorax	• Shortness of breath	Chest tube
Aspiration	• Cough, pneumonia • Change in color of secretions	Cannot occur with a laryngectomy (unless pharyngo-stomal fistula) Reflux precautions, improved airway care, antibiotics

can be described as throbbing head pressure related to the intracranial rise in spinal fluid pressure that occurs when the jugular vein is sacrificed. Because of the resection of nerve roots of C 2-3-4, the sensory branches supplying the skin of the neck and scalp, incisional pain is somewhat mediated and better controlled with medications. Patients requiring a skin graft often complain that the donor site on the thigh is more painful than the head and neck incision. The use of hydrophilic dressings will markedly decrease the amount of pain experienced at the donor site.

Head and neck surgery often results in alterations in speaking, limiting the patient's ability to describe the pain and response to interventions. Signs and symptoms of postoperative pain unique to the patient with head and neck cancer include facial grimacing, squinting, elevated shoulders, limited or no movement of the upper torso, bracing, restlessness, glabellar frowning, and shoulder and neck stiffness (Feldt, 2000). Adequate pain control promotes comfort and encourages early ambulation and coughing and deep breathing to clear secretions.

Manage acute postoperative pain with the administration of opioids for several days. Alternating morphine and acetaminophen with codeine has been proven to be effective in controlling early postoperative pain (Cherny, 2000). An alternative to intermittent dosing in the early postoperative period is the use of patient-controlled analgesia. For the narcotic- or opiate-naïve patient, the dosing schedule should be a consistent administration plan with as-needed dosing for breakthrough pain (Cherny). Aggressive nursing care focuses on patient comfort during the first 24–48 hours following surgery. When opioids are no longer required, nonopioid analgesics may be administered by enteral routes. Administer medications in liquid form or crush and administer through the feeding tube. The feeding tube must be flushed after administration of the analgesic to prevent obstruction of the tube (Bockus, 1991).

Other concerns in the management of pain in the patient with cancer of the head and neck are age, comorbidities that may affect the medication requirements, and length of surgery with associated positioning. Many patients with head and neck cancer are older adults, presenting with the age-related pain of arthritis (American Geriatrics Society, 1998). Even for younger adults, positioning during a lengthy surgery and postoperative bedrest contributes to immobility, with associated pain relieved by the administration of adequate pain medication and early ambulation (American Pain Society [APS], 1995, 1999). Nurses must balance analgesic administration against the patient's hemodynamic and respiratory conditions, the medical plan and prescriptions, and the desires of the patient and family (Stannard et al., 1996).

As the patient recovers from surgery, the need for pain medication decreases. Useful drugs include acetaminophen, acetaminophen with codeine, and nonsteroidal anti-inflammatory drugs (Cherny, 2000). Some individuals will benefit from the use of a fentanyl transdermal patch or, if the oral route is possible, an extended-release oral morphine. This regimen provides adequate pain relief without interruption of activities of daily living and results in better sleep (APS, 1995). Consultation with a pain service can offer alternative medications and supportive therapies (Miaskowski, Crews, Ready, Paul, & Ginsberg, 1999).

Supportive Pain Therapy

Postoperative pain relief following cancer surgery is an example of palliative care. Palliative care has been defined as the relief and prevention of suffering. Suffering has four components: physical, psychological, social, and spiritual (Meyers & Linder, 2003). For the physical pain, consider the use of nonpharmacologic supportive therapy for pain management. For example, a physical therapy consultation to institute exercises to improve ambulation, facial muscle relaxation, deep breathing, positioning, and safety also may provide pain relief. If the patient complains of masseter or jaw pain, offer instruction for exercises to clench and unclench the jaws, open the mouth, and massage the temporal fossa. Following neck dissection, physical therapy for range of motion and massage and relaxation exercises for the trapezius muscle will provide relief of pain in this area (Patt, 1990).

Approximately 70%–90% of pain resulting from cancer can be relieved relatively simply with oral analgesics and adjuvant drugs in accordance with the World Health Organization's (1996) guidelines. The remaining 10%–30% can be difficult to treat. Adjuvant medications, such as antidepressants, anticonvulsants, nonsteroidal anti-inflammatory drugs, steroids, local and topical pain agents, antianxiety agents, and neuropathic agents, are helpful additions to the pain management protocol (Sykes, Johnson, & Hanks, 1997).

Wound Management

Patients with head and neck cancer are at risk for impaired wound healing because of malnutrition, preoperative radiation therapy, and smoking. A low serum albumin, < 2.0 g/dl, is associated with decreased tensile strength and poor wound healing. Preoperative radiation therapy increases the risk of delayed healing because of vascular impairment and impaired cellular nutrition. Also consider the smoking-related issues of vascular disease, particularly peripheral vascular disease with impaired circulation (van Bokhorst-de van der Schueren et al., 1999). Wound management begins with an initial postoperative assessment (see Table 9-3). Assess the suture lines every three to four hours, noting the color, temperature, and adequacy of blood supply. Flaps should be pink in color, feel warm to the touch, and have good capillary refill. A cool, bluish or dusky flap indicates venous congestion and the presence

Table 9-3. University of California, Davis Medical Center Ear, Nose, and Throat (ENT) Intensive Care Unit Matrix for the Care of Patients With Head and Neck Cancer

	Topic	Site	Nursing Interventions	Frequency
1	Airway	Tracheostomy	• Temporary airway • Cuff inflated while on ventilator • Always check cuff pressures • Cuff deflated at all other times • Position by securing from shoulders (not chest) Stomahesive® and Elastoplast® (Beiersdorf, Hamburg, Germany). • No ties over reconstruction flaps or grafts • Instill saline frequently suction prn • Tracheostomy wound care • Spare tube at bedside	Q shift and prn Q 2 hours and prn Q 4–8 hours and prn
		Laryngectomy	• Permanent airway trachea sutured to anterior skin of neck • Stoma care: cotton swabs with hydrogen peroxide and normal saline • Remove crusts over suture lines • Instill saline frequently suction prn • Goal is shiny glistening mucosa in airway. • Bayonet forceps at bedside for secretion removal • Stoma button if stoma contracts • If tracheoesophageal puncture (TEP), secure tube and alternate left to right side. • May feed via TEP if in stomach.	Q 2 hours and prn Q 2–4 hours and prn Q shift and prn Q 2–4 hours and prn
2	Nutrition	Oral, nasogastric (NG), gastrostomy tube, jejunostomy tube, or via TEP	• Do not move NG tube. • Secure with Stomahesive and tape to nares. • Do not remove nasal stitch. • Do not attempt to replace NG without physician order. • Administer feedings by nutrition consult. • Chyle leak—feed only nonfat formula (Vivonex® [Novartis, East Hanover, NJ] T.E.N. or similar).	Change and clean prn Continuous then bolus
3	Drains	Varidyne® (Sterion, Minneapolis, MN) suction vacuum pump or Jackson-Pratt® (Cardinal Health, Dublin, OH) drain	• Secure with Stomahesive and Elastoplast. • Strip to prevent clots. • Strict output recording • Call house officer if sudden increase or decrease in output or air leaks. • Pressure dressing for 24 hours after drain removal	Q 1–2 hours

4	Flaps	• Myocutaneous
		• Microvascular free flap
		• Radial forearm
		• Fibula
		• Rectus
		• Scapula
		• Rotation flap
			• Color
			  - Venous congestion = red
			  - No arterial supply = white
			• Capillary refill
			• No pressure by lines, drains, or tapes
			• Doppler for arterial and/or venous pulse
			• Keep blood pressure stable at all times to keep microvascular and pedicle vessels patent.
				Q 1–2 hours and prn
				
				Q 1–2 hours and prn
				
				Q 1–2 hours and prn

5	Wound Care	Head and neck incisions	• Use hydrogen peroxide to remove crusts. • Apply light antibiotic ointment to prevent crusts (first three days only).	Q 1–2 hours and prn
		Split-thickness skin graft/full thickness skin graft (usually on thigh)	• Change hydrogel (or similar) (**not** Xeroform). • When no longer painful during change, leave open to air. Postoperative days 5–7	Q day and prn

(Continued on next page)

Table 9-3. University of California, Davis Medical Center Ear, Nose, and Throat (ENT) Intensive Care Unit Matrix for the Care of Patients With Head and Neck Cancer (Continued)

	Topic	Site	Nursing Interventions	Frequency

		Free flap donor site	• Do not change dressings.
			• Check neurovascular status—movement, sensation, capillary refill, temperature.
			  - Radial forearm free flap → fingers
			  - Fibular free flap → toes
				Q 2 hours advancing to Q 4 hours; then as ordered

6	Fistula	• Orocutaneous • Pharyngocutane-ous	• Dressing wet to dry, open fluffs and pack carefully. • Protect airway.	Q 2 hours then Q 4 hours and prn
7	Carotid	• Internal carotid artery • Exposed external or intraoral	• Wet-to-wet to keep carotid in a wet and clean environment • Hetastarch in sodium chloride at bedside • Type and cross (or hold) two units. • Two large-bore IVs • Alert operating room that patient is on precautions. • If bleed occurs, apply direct pressure and do not remove. • Call ENT resident on call for emergency intervention. • If healing, wet with saline, alternating with dressing changes.	Q 2 hours around the clock (ATC) and prn Give volume expanders, continue pressure, secure airway, and transport to operating room with surgeon. Q 2 hours, then Q 4 hours; wet with saline in between.
8	Pain	Post-op management	• Regular frequent dosing of opioids • Acetaminophen with codeine (or similar) alternating • Acetaminophen with codeine for caffeine withdrawal headaches • Do not sedate if inadequately medicated for pain. • Always check for previous pain medication use—do not assume opiate-naïve. • If patients' pain is well managed in ICU, they generally require less pain medication on general ENT floor. • Routine bowel care	Q 1–2 hours for the first 24 hours, then prn but ATC; assess frequently according to pain guidelines.
9	ETOH (alcohol) with-drawal	–	• Regular dosing of benzodiazepines • Use agitation protocol judiciously. • Continue pain medication. • Psych/social consults and behavior modification	Restraints for safety prn
10	Patient teaching	Consistent plan according to policy and patient educa-tion records	• Begin pre-op, continue post-op and into clinic • Ongoing teaching • Reevaluation necessary • Documentation	Ongoing

Note. Copyright 2003 by Ann E.F. Sievers, University of California, Davis Medical Center. Reprinted with permission.

of a hematoma. Detailed documentation of the wound status, augmented by pictures or diagrams, assists in monitoring the wound (see Table 9-3).

The postoperative head and neck surgery patient may have both internal and external incisions. Standard incision care includes cleaning the suture line with hydrogen peroxide to remove crusts and normal saline. Antibiotic ointment is applied to the incision during the first few days after surgery. Correct positioning of the patient will prevent tension on the wound and vascular compression of the flaps from drains, ventilator tubing, and tracheostomy ties (Sigler, 1988).

Drains

Multiple drains are placed during surgery to remove blood and serum, seal the skin flaps to the underlying wound bed, and prevent hematoma formation (Sievers, 1984). Drains must be secure at all times to prevent inadvertent removal (see Table 9-3). The integrity of the drains is critical to wound healing. Strip the drains every one to two hours to prevent obstruction by clots and to maintain patency. The drainage should be monitored each shift, noting the color, amount, and consistency of drainage (Clarke, 1998). In the presence of multiple drains, each drain should be labeled as to its location to permit documentation of output and to guide drain removal.

Any sudden change in the amount of drainage may indicate hematoma or seroma formation, resulting in a compromise of the vascular bed. Drainage initially is sanguineous but changes to serosanguineous and then serous drainage within a few days. Surgical drains remain in place until output is less than 25 cc in a 24-hour period and usually are removed at postoperative day three to six (Sigler & Schuring, 1993). Following drain removal, a pressure dressing placed over the incision prevents reaccumulation of fluid under the flap. This dressing usually is in place for 24 hours.

Edema

Head and neck surgery often causes edema of the face and neck resulting from removal of lymphatic channels and resection of the jugular vein during neck dissection, both of which impede drainage. Postoperative edema can be significant, and supportive measures are necessary to minimize swelling. Elevate the head of the bed and avoid constricting clothing and tracheostomy ties. Edema of the head and neck usually peaks three to five days after mobilization of intra/extravascular fluid and recedes after two to six months (Cutright & Guadagnini, 1998). During the postoperative flux of fluid shifts, electrolytes, particularly serum sodium and potassium, should be monitored. Both are influential in maintaining cellular integrity and managing postoperative edema (van Bokhorst-de van der Schueren et al., 2000).

Significant edema may interfere with sensory function and is frightening to both the patient and family. Periorbital edema impairs vision; neck edema may impair speech and mobility of the neck; and eustachian tube edema decreases hearing (Harris, 1998). Explaining the rationale for the swelling and offering supportive measures to decrease the edema may alleviate some anxiety. Adequate pain control and the use of antianxiety medications may also help the patient.

Cerebral edema may result following radical neck dissection (especially bilateral) and skull base surgery. Cerebral edema is manifested by an alteration in the level of consciousness, confusion, and delirium. Alcohol withdrawal and medication delirium also may occur simultaneously (see Table 9-3).

Flaps and Grafts

Split thickness skin grafts often are used to resurface oral cavity resections when large amounts of tissue and bone are not required. A thin layer of skin from the anterior thigh is removed and placed over the wound. The donor site is painful because of the exposure of the superficial nerve fibers. Placing a hydrocolloid dressing over the wound to protect the area markedly decreases the pain and improves wound healing. The dressing over the graft donor site remains in place for five to seven days. Once the dressing has been removed, it can be changed daily until the site is no longer painful. At this time, the donor site is exposed to the air to permit healing. Once completely healed, the scar tissue over the graft donor site can be massaged (Wiechula, 2003).

Immediate reconstruction of the surgical defect usually is performed at the time of tumor resection. Surgical reconstruction techniques include primary closure, rotation flaps, muscle and skin transfers (myocutaneous flaps), and free tissue transfers. Myocutaneous flaps used for reconstruction of head and neck defects include pectoralis major myocutaneous flaps, skinless pectoralis flaps, and other flaps designed to repair the defect created by the tumor resection. Microvascular free flaps also are used for reconstruction and require specific expertise by physicians as well as nurses. Commonly used free flap sites include the radial forearm, fibula, scapula, and rectus muscle. Specific considerations depend on the site selected. For example, the patient is not permitted any weight bearing for 7–10 days when the fibula is used for reconstruction, and the nondominant arm usually is selected as the donor site when a radial forearm free flap is used.

Regardless of the donor site used (arm, leg, or back), similar nursing assessment and interventions are followed during the immediate postoperative period. A Doppler sound device assesses the microvascular anastomosis for patency. Doppler the site every hour. If the blood flow by Doppler is stable and the reconstruction flap maintains a pink color after the first three days, the assessment can take place every four to six hours, progressing to every shift until discharge. A stable blood pressure, with a mean arterial pressure of approximately 60–80 mm Hg, is necessary to sustain blood flow through the vascular pedicle. IV dextran and/or aspirin prevent clotting at the anastomosis site. Extremity donor sites should have neurovascular assessments each hour. Assess the fingers (radial forearm free flap) or the toes (fibular free flap) for color, temperature, and ability to sense touch and to move on command (Devine, Potter, Magennis, Brown, & Vaughan, 2001).

Physical therapy and occupational therapy are consulted for patients who have undergone free flap reconstruction. Direct each therapy to the disability from the resections and the reconstruction, such as stability in ambulation after fibula grafts, hand range of motion after forearm flaps, and shoulder exercises after neck dissection. Shoulder exercises are necessary after resection of cranial nerve XI (spinal accessory) with neck dissection. Each center will establish specific protocols for monitoring and therapy (Devine et al., 2001).

All flaps should be assessed for color, temperature, and integrity. Bulging of the flap, increase in drain output, fullness of the flap, and color changes may be signs of vascular compromise and must be reported immediately to the reconstruction surgeon. Significant changes in the flap may require additional surgery to decompress the vascular compromise, artery, or vein.

Eye Care

Following temporal bone dissection, parotidectomy, or extensive ear surgery, the function of the facial nerve must be evaluated. The facial nerve, cranial nerve VII, may be resected or injured, resulting in a temporary or permanent paresis. Each of the five branches of the nerve is important to the structure and function of the facial musculature. If the patient is unable to fully close the eye, the cornea is exposed to drying air with resultant corneal abrasion. A protocol for eye care should be started for anyone with facial nerve dysfunction. If the cornea is visible with the dysfunction or the blink is absent, the patient should instill lubricating eye drops every two hours and apply an ointment at bedtime. The patient also should wear a clear eye shield or tape the eye closed while sleeping. Eye care continues until the facial nerve function returns or surgery is performed to insert a gold weight in the upper eyelid to allow for closure.

Oral Care

Oral cavity resections create an exposed intraoral suture line. Good oral care is essential to stimulate blood supply, promote healing, reduce edema, prevent infection, control odors, and alleviate pain and discomfort (Munro & Grap, 2004). Carefully cleanse the oral cavity with normal saline and chlorhexidine solution, as ordered, using soft brushes or brush and suction devices. Special care is necessary to avoid injury to the suture line. Good lighting is essential to inspect the intraoral tissues and assess the integrity of the suture line.

Postsurgical Complications

Postoperative Hemorrhage

The most common cause of hemorrhage in the early postoperative period is ligature slippage. But regardless of the cause, the nurse must be observant to standard signs and symptoms of postoperative hemorrhage. This includes tense and bulging flaps, expansion of the flap, oozing at the suture line, drop in blood pressure, restlessness, possibly hypoxia, and blood in the surgical drains. Because each drain is placed in a specific anatomic area, increased bleeding from an individual drain helps to locate the area of bleeding.

If any of the aforementioned signs and symptoms occurs, the nurse and the surgeon must be in constant contact and evaluate the patient together. Bleeding at the wound bed often necessitates a prompt return to surgery to explore the wound,

control the bleeding, and save the reconstruction flaps (Devine et al., 2001).

Chyle Leak

The appearance of copious amounts of milky white, opaque drainage may indicate the presence of a chyle fistula. This is an infrequent complication caused by a leak from the thoracic duct into the lateral neck wound, usually following a left neck dissection. The drainage is analyzed for the presence of amylase. Chyle fistulas are managed conservatively with nonfat diets, observation for fluid and electrolyte imbalance, and the placement of a pressure dressing over the anterior chest. With time and a decrease in the flow of chyle production because of the nonfat diet, the leak may heal itself. If the fistula does not close, surgical intervention to close the opening may be needed. If the drainage is not recognized as chyle, depletion of total body protein and fluid and electrolyte imbalances may occur (McCray & Parrish, 2004).

Fistula

A fistula is a breakdown of a suture line creating communication between two sites, such as the oral cavity and the neck (orocutaneous fistula) or the pharynx and the neck (pharyngocutaneous fistula). A fistula usually is apparent three to five days postoperatively and occurs because of a disruption of a surgical incision. Causes of a fistula include poor nutrition, prior radiation therapy, and contamination of the wound. Symptoms include a low-grade fever (100–101°F), drainage, confusion, tachycardia, erythema and tenderness of the suture line, or purulence (Cutright & Guadagnini, 1998).

The standard of care is to open the suture line widely to facilitate drainage, debride the wound, pack the wound with sterile wet dressings to promote granulation and healing, and administer IV antibiotics. Diversion of the salivary stream away from the wound and the airway facilitates wound healing. The use of a tonsil-tip oral suction device helps to control the saliva. The patient is NPO and receives enteral feedings to prevent food from entering the wound while still providing good nutrition. Pain medication and topical anesthetic agents may be used to minimize the pain associated with dressing changes and debridement. A fistula heals naturally, from the wound bed outward. Once granulation tissue is established in the wound, the patient and/or family may be taught how to change the dressing in preparation for home care.

Carotid Artery Rupture

Rupture of the common carotid artery is a life-threatening oncologic emergency. Nurses must be aware of the risk factors, signs, and symptoms and establish a consistent, standard plan of care (see Table 9-3). Exposure of the carotid artery can occur because of wound infection and necrosis, dehiscence of the wound over the carotid artery, tumor infiltration, or flap failure with a fistula. Exposure of the carotid artery results in weakening of the artery with the potential for rupture (Schiech, 2000). The two most common risk factors for exposure of the artery or rupture are destruction of the carotid vascular supply because of previous radiation therapy and devascularization of the carotid artery during neck dissection (Steele et al., 2004). Carotid exposure can occur externally through the neck or internally from the oropharynx. An internal bleed is much more difficult to control because of limited access to the bleeding site.

The overall goal is to prevent drying of the carotid adventitia, the outermost layer of the artery. The adventitia dries and forms an eschar. If the eschar is disrupted, hemorrhage will occur. A small sentinel bleed may precede arterial rupture and must be reported immediately because surgical intervention is indicated to stop the bleeding. High epigastric pain also may indicate impending hemorrhage. The patient exhibits pain because the shearing forces in the artery destroy the fibers of the vagus nerve (cranial nerve X). This sensory pathway accounts for the symptom of pain (Schwartz & Barr, 1979).

The patient who is at risk for carotid artery rupture is placed on "carotid precautions," and emergency supplies are placed at the bedside. Emergency supplies include dressings, IV sets of fluid and volume expanders, artificial airways, and syringes to inflate the tracheostomy cuff. The patient should occupy a room close to the nursing station to allow for constant observation. The nurse should monitor vital signs, airway, responsiveness, and pain. IV access is maintained with a wide-bore IV to allow for immediate infusion of fluids and blood in the event of rupture. Wound care includes gentle packing of the wound with saline-soaked nonadhering dressings to keep the exposed carotid artery moist and the wound bed clean. Wet-to-wet dressings are changed every two hours. Dressing changes advance to every four hours, and normal saline solution is applied every two hours between dressing changes as the wound heals. This also will provide a longer period of uninterrupted sleep for the patient.

In the event of carotid artery rupture, aggressive, immediate treatment is paramount to saving the patient's life. The nurse must remain with the patient and immediately apply digital pressure to the carotid. Dressings that allow direct point pressure to the site of the rupture should be used. Avoid use of bulky dressings, which impair the ability to localize the site of bleeding. Inflate the cuff immediately to seal the airway if an artificial airway is in place. IV fluid or a volume expander is infused rapidly to prevent hypovolemic shock. Maintain pressure over the carotid until surgery is available to manage the bleeding. The patient is prepared for transport to the operating room for vessel ligation. Postligation, the patient should be observed for neurologic deficits or signs of stroke from cerebral hypoxia (Schiech, 2000).

Early determination must be made regarding the patient's wishes in the event of a carotid artery rupture. This discussion must occur as soon as the exposed artery is identified. In the face of recurrent, untreatable cancer, some patients request no intervention. Death is very quick from a carotid artery rupture; however, it is traumatic for anyone attending to the patient, including family and healthcare providers. Everyone, especially the patient, must be prepared for the event. In many cases, the patient will remain conscious throughout the event and should be cared for with sensitivity and support. In the hospital setting, dark green scrub towels are kept at the bedside, and at home, dark towels are recommended to minimize the visual effect of a large blood loss. Hospice or home health nurses must continue the conversation about the patient's wishes and preferred action if a carotid artery rupture occurs (Pereira & Phan, 2004). A debriefing session is valuable to support the staff following this traumatic event. Consultation with a social worker or psychiatric liaison also may be helpful.

Cranial Nerve and Neurologic Impairment

Following head and neck surgery, neurologic impairment may result from either tumor involvement, surgical resection, or perioperative hypotension Symptoms include delirium, dementia, depression, cranial nerve dysfunction, and vascular impairment resulting in stroke. An accurate preoperative assessment is crucial to establish a baseline for comparison because the patient may have preexisting dementia or depression or suffered previous strokes (Andresen et al., 1998).

In the immediate postoperative period, assess cranial nerves and cognitive function (see Table 9-4). Administration of the Mini-Mental State Examination (Folstein, Folstein, & McHugh, 1975) or any similar test and a good neurologic and physiologic exam can detect impairments (Andresen et al., 1998). A complete evaluation of the cognitive function may be limited because of the patient's inability to speak, but cognitive function also can be assessed by reviewing the patient's written responses for context, spelling, organization, and correct answers (Fuller, 1993).

Nutritional Management

Patients with head and neck cancer often are malnourished at the time of diagnosis because of the tumor and the tumor-associated symptoms of dysphagia and odynophagia. Patients complain of chewing and swallowing difficulties that result in decreased oral intake with subsequent weight loss and cachexia. Poor dietary habits also result from a history of alcohol and tobacco abuse and can lead to changes in metabolism and vitamin and mineral deficiencies, which further contribute to malnutrition. Maintenance of proper nutrition throughout the perioperative experience is crucial to the healing process and recovery (van Bokhorst-de van der Schueren et al., 1999, 2000).

Table 9-4. University of California, Davis Medical Center Cranial Nerve Impairments Nursing and Patient Issues

Cranial Nerve	Name	Cause or Reason for Impairment	Target	Nursing and Patient Issues
I	Olfactory *Sensory*	• Rhinectomy • Anterior skull base tumor • Laryngectomy	• Olfactory bulb	• Safety issues resulting from loss of smell
II	Optic *Sensory*	• Resection • Tumor, stroke	• Eye	• Blindness
III	Oculomotor *Motor*	• Anterior cranial facial resection • Tumor, stroke	• Eye movement	• Visual field limitations
IV	Trochlear *Motor*	• Anterior cranial facial resection • Tumor, stroke	• Eye movement	• Visual field limitations
V	Trigeminal *Sensory* *Motor*	• Anterior cranial facial resection • Tumor, stroke	• Muscles of mastication	• Numbness, so decreased postoperative pain
VI	Abducent *Motor*	• Anterior cranial facial resection • Tumor, stroke	• Eye movement	• Visual field limitations
VII	Facial *Motor*	• Temporal bone resection • Acoustic neuroma • Parotidectomy	• Five branches for facial movement/oral competence	• Eye protection and safety drops • Lubrication at night • Moisture chamber • Oral drooling
VII	Facial Chorda tympani *Sensory*	• Temporal bone resection • Acoustic neuroma • Parotidectomy	• Taste (anterior two-thirds of the tongue)	• Pleasure and safety
VIII	Acoustic or vestibulocochlear *Sensory* Cochlear Vestibular	• Acoustic neuroma • Lateral skull base • Lateral temporal bone	• Hearing • Balance	• Hearing • Safety and balance issues
IX	Glossopharyngeal *Motor* *Sensory*	• Base of tongue • Laryngectomy	• Taste (posterior third of the tongue)	• Pleasure • Safety
X	Vagus *Motor* *Sensory*	• Resection of recurrent laryngeal nerve, superior laryngeal nerve	• Vocal function • Sensation of the larynx	• Airway, speech • Oral nutrition without aspiration
XI	Spinal accessory *Motor*	• Radical neck dissection	• Paralysis of the trapezius • "Winging" of the scapula • Frozen shoulder	• Physical therapy • Compliance with exercises • Prevention of frozen shoulder
XII	Hypoglossal *Motor*	• Base of tongue resection	• Speech and swallowing	• Speech therapy • Safety in nutrition
C 2-3-4	Cervical plexus *Sensory*	–	• Numbness in ear • Scalp sensitivity • Supraclavicular numbness	• No feeling for injury • Pain on combing hair

Note. Copyright 2002 by Ann E.F. Sievers, University of California, Davis Medical Center. Reprinted with permission.

The patient with head and neck cancer has a functional gastrointestinal tract that allows for enteral feeding. The patient with head and neck cancer also has a significant insensible water loss caused by suctioning of the mouth and artificial airway. This requires special attention to fluid replacement along with nutrition replacement. Improvement of the patient's nutritional state is a challenge that requires a multidisciplinary approach for optimal success.

Early intervention begins with a preoperative baseline nutritional assessment by a clinical dietitian to develop a nutritional plan of care. The medical, nursing, nutrition, and medication history, physical examination, anthropometric measurements, and laboratory data are all used to develop a nutritional plan of care. Screening tools such as the Nutrition Screening Initiative Checklist (www.aafp.org/nsi.xml) and the Hydration Assessment Checklist from the Hartford Institute for Geriatric Nursing (www.hartfordign.org/pdf/TTnutrition.pdf) may be helpful. Objective measurements include height, weight, pre-illness weight, weight change over time, and body mass index.

Postoperatively, the patient will be NPO until edema subsides, suture lines are healed, and the patient demonstrates the ability to swallow without aspiration. The patient will receive enteral therapy during this time to prevent stress on the suture lines and reduce the risk of aspiration. The choice and location of the enteral feeding tube are critical to the method of feeding. A small-bore nasogastric tube (NGT) is used for short-term feedings (less than seven days). A gastrostomy tube (GT) is preferable for the patient who will require long-term enteral support as well as postoperative radiation therapy. A jejunostomy tube (JT) is selected when a GT is contraindicated and for the patient who has had gastric procedures. Surgically placed tubes result in discomfort at the site for several days. Administer pain medication as needed and assist the patient with positioning and mobility until the pain subsides. Assess the tube site daily for the presence of drainage and skin breakdown. Clean the site with half-strength hydrogen peroxide to remove crusting. Use a gauze dressing if the area is draining (Arbogast, 2002).

Administer NGT and GT feedings by bolus or continuous feedings, as tolerated by the patient. Deliver JT feedings continuously to prevent dumping syndrome. Patients restarting nutrition with high-carbohydrate feedings after a prolonged period of malnutrition are at risk for refeeding syndrome or metabolic and physiologic changes that may result in hyperglycemia and fluid overload and should be monitored closely (Ladage, 2003). The refeeding syndrome occurs in patients who are chronically semistarved or marasmic. These patients have adapted to the use of free fatty acids and ketone bodies as energy sources. Refeeding can result in metabolic abnormalities, including hypophosphatemia, hypokalemia, and hypomagnesemia. Patient symptoms are cardiac, neuromuscular and respiratory dysfunction, and fluid retention (ASPEN Board of Directors & The Clinical Guidelines Task Force, 2002). Monitor glucose, phosphorus, potassium, and magnesium until levels are normal.

Enteral therapy begins on postoperative day one or two. Most feedings are initiated when bowel sounds are heard, although current thought indicates that if the gut is intact, feeding may begin prior to the resumption of bowel sounds (Cheever, 1999). Prior to the administration of feedings, verify the placement of the feeding tube and check for residual feedings by aspirating gastric contents (Arbogast, 2002). The choice of nutritional support for enteral feeding is based on caloric density, protein, fiber, osmolality, and fluid needs (see Figure 9-5). Continuous, slow feedings are initiated using a feeding pump, and the volume and rate are gradually increased. The patient may advance to a bolus feeding as tolerated. Administer feedings three to four times daily, similar to normal meal times. Smaller feedings can be considered for those patients who have slight to moderate intolerance to larger quantities.

Weigh the patient on a regular schedule and record weights to determine progress. Documentation of caloric intake as well as fluid intake and output is necessary to ensure adequacy of the feeding regimen. Monitor the patient closely for complications and intolerance problems. Potential complications of enteral feedings include blockage of the tube and signs of intolerance, such as fullness, nausea and vomiting, and dumping syndrome. If intolerance occurs, decrease the amount and strength of feeding and consult a dietitian for further recommendations, as the patient is at nutritional risk (ASPEN Board of Directors & The Clinical Guidelines Task Force, 2002).

Aspiration is of particular concern for the patient following head and neck surgery. Monitor the patient for any signs of aspiration. In the past, a blue dye was placed in tube feedings to detect aspiration. This practice recently has been scrutinized. Studies have shown that blue food dye may act as an inhibitor of oxidative phosphorylation in the cell mitochondria. Limited phosphorylation may inhibit mitochondria respiration, potentially resulting in complications such as hypotension, acidosis, and death (Maloney et al., 2000).

Figure 9-5. Targets for Nutritional Goals for Postsurgical Head and Neck Cancer Patients— Estimated Macronutrient Guidelines

- Protein: 1.0–1.5 pro/kg reference weight
- Water: 27–35 ml/kg or 1 ml water/kcal
- Vitamins and minerals: Recommended daily allowance requirements
- Calories: 28–33 calories/kg reference weight

Reference weight
- Females: 100 lbs first 5 feet + 5 lbs for each additional inch
- Males: 106 lbs first 5 feet + 6 lbs for each additional inch

Note. Copyright 2003 by Beverly Lorens, University of California, Davis Medical Center. Reprinted with permission.

To prepare for home enteral feeding, teach the patient and family to administer the feedings. Supervise the administration of feedings until the patient and family are proficient.

Swallowing

Excision of a tumor of the head and neck may result in a surgical defect with loss of structures that can result in difficulty in swallowing. The method of reconstruction will subsequently influence the character and the severity of the dysphagia and degree of aspiration. Swallowing defects may occur in any of the four phases of swallowing: oral preparatory, oral, pharyngeal, and esophageal (Logemann, 1997). When radiation therapy is added to the regimen postoperatively, dysphagia may worsen secondary to xerostomia and soft tissue fibrosis in the field of radiation exposure (Kendall, McKenzie, Leonard, & Jones, 1998).

A postoperative goal is to maintain nutrition for wound healing and protect the airway from aspiration while rehabilitating the patient's ability to swallow an oral diet. If oral nutrition is not possible, safe methods of "social nutrition" may be explored. Maintain the patient's nutrition by enteral feeding methods, such as GT feedings. After performing a swallow assessment by a dynamic swallowing study (DSS), define methods by which the patient can safely take oral nutrition. These methods may include the patient consuming controlled amounts (½–1 teaspoon) of selected liquids or solids while in specific positions (head turned, chin tucked, side lying) that allow the patient to safely take limited food without the risk of aspiration. Even these small amounts may allow the person to enjoy favorite foods at the dining table with family for "social nutrition." Patients who are weak generally lack sufficient breath support and have a poor cough in response to airway penetration by food or liquid, making them less able to respond effectively to even mild aspiration. Early identification of patients with dysphagia is important to prevent nutritional and aspiration-related complications (Sievers, 1997).

Patients who have undergone total laryngectomy cannot aspirate because of the surgical disconnection of the trachea and the digestive tract. Patients who have undergone composite resections for oral cavity tumors are at higher risk for aspiration because of the alteration of the oral cavity and the presence of an intact and vulnerable larynx (see Figures 9-6 and 9-7). Aspiration is diagnosed based on the following parameters: (a) the signs and symptoms of infection, including fever, tachycardia, tachypnea, increased white blood cell count, decreased breath sounds, and respiratory failure; (b) radiographic changes, including consolidation, infiltration, and elevated hemidiaphragm; (c) bacterial cultures from sputum; and (d) hypoxemia based on arterial blood gases and pulse oximetry results (Metheny, Aud, & Wunderlich, 1999).

Figure 9-6. Risk Factors for Aspiration

- Decreased level of consciousness
- Supine position
- Presence of a nasogastric tube
- Tracheal intubation and mechanical ventilation
- Bolus or intermittent feeding delivery methods
- Malpositioned feeding tube
- Vomiting
- High-risk disease and injury conditions
- Neurologic disorders
- Major abdominal and thoracic trauma/surgery
- Diabetes mellitus
- Poor oral health
- Inadequate RN staffing levels
- Advanced age

Note. Based on information from Metheny, 2002.

Figure 9-7. Methods for Decreasing Risk of Aspiration Pneumonia in Critically Ill Patients

- Adjust body position.
- Administer kinetic bed therapy.
- Change method of formula delivery and size of nasogastric tube.
- Administer gastric pH specialized formulas and medications.
- Suction subglottic secretions.
- Perform oral and selective digestive bacterial decontamination.

Note. Based on information from Scolapio, 2002.

Swallowing Evaluation

A speech-language pathologist trained in the care of patients with head and neck cancer should perform a swallowing evaluation. The goals of the evaluation are to gain objective information about the patient's swallowing, to assess the patient's ability to sustain oral nutrition, to protect the airway, and to determine methods for rehabilitation. The assessment includes a complete history (medical, surgical, and nutritional), physical examination (including anatomic and cranial nerve evaluation), flexible endoscopic evaluation including examination of the laryngeal function and sensation, clinical swallowing examination, and, if indicated, a dynamic radiograph of the swallow and DSS (Logemann, 1997).

The clinical swallowing examination does not allow visualization of the entire swallowing tract and thus cannot provide certain information regarding oral, pharyngeal, and laryngeal structures and function. It cannot provide definitive information about whether a patient is aspirating or why aspiration is occurring. It is not meant to be a substitute for the current gold standard of dysphagia assessment, the DSS (Goodrich & Walker, 1997). This assessment includes behavioral observations of the patient's ability to clear the oral cavity; cough; clear the airway before, during, and after the swallow; voicing before and after swallowing; respiration sounds; elevation of laryngeal structures; laryngeal auscultation; and evidence of struggle (Goodrich & Walker). Clinical evaluations also include cranial nerve assessments and breath support. A thorough understanding of the surgical procedure and reconstruction is paramount to understanding the reasons for swallowing impairment.

The DSS is the most objective of all evaluations. The DSS includes timing with quantitative measurements by addressing postsurgical structure, function, and airway integrity. It also provides information about the patient's response to strategies used during therapy. The plan for swallowing therapy can only be determined by obtaining accurate information. Rehabilitation of the patient's normal swallow is crucial to the patient's recovery, but it should never be at the expense of the maintenance of adequate nutrition (McKenzie, 1997).

Communication

"But the most traumatic result of the surgery was the loss of voice, even though I had known it was coming. My doctor had said that . . . it is more shattering to the patient than coming out of an operation blind" (Dresden, 1978, p. 46).

The alterations to communication following head and neck surgery pose a unique challenge to most patients. Preoperative teaching by both the nurse and the speech-language pathologist about the loss of normal communication, even if temporary, is essential to postoperative adaptation and recovery.

The nurse should discuss the inability to communicate by voice and offer the patient and family options for postoperative communication, including the use of pads and pencils, dry-erase boards, and magic slates. The patient's ability, method, and preferences for communication need to be assessed, and the patient's ability to read and write also should be evaluated because approximately 48% of Americans are functionally illiterate (Kirsch, Jungeblut, Jenkins, & Kolstad, 1993). Knowledge of the patient's native language and level of education also is essential. The speech-language pathologist evaluates the patient's ability to articulate and use facial communication and hand gestures. Patients who are more naturally animated speakers usually will cope and communicate better after surgery.

The type of head and neck surgical procedure performed will determine the type of communication change that the patient can anticipate. Patients who have had an oral cavity resection usually will have a temporary loss of voice until the tracheostomy is removed and may have problems with articulation. Speech therapy is indicated, and the patient will require exercises to increase strength, range of motion, and coordination of the tongue.

A laryngectomy affects the patient's ability to phonate and can be further divided into voice preservation for partial laryngectomy candidates or total laryngectomy voice ablation candidates. These patients *must* work with a speech-language pathologist trained in total and partial laryngectomy therapy.

Alternate communication techniques include written, prewritten, computer-generated, and artificial devices. Patients who undergo laryngectomy have multiple choices for communication and use different methods in different situations. Communication options include the use of an electrolarynx, tracheoesophageal puncture with voice prosthesis, esophageal speech, and a combination of all methods (see Figure 9-8).

Understanding the patient's specific needs is essential in supporting postoperative communication. The nurse must take the time to listen and understand an individual's speech pattern and focus on articulation as well as context. The investment of time and patience will result in patient confidence and appreciation.

Body Image Disturbance

Body image is the unique perception each person has of his or her own body in terms of physical appearance, function, and emotional reactions (Dropkin, 1997). Surgical treatment for cancer of the head and neck may involve radical resections of soft tissue and bone from the face and neck, resulting

Figure 9-8. Anatomy of a Total Neck Breather With Tracheoesophageal Puncture

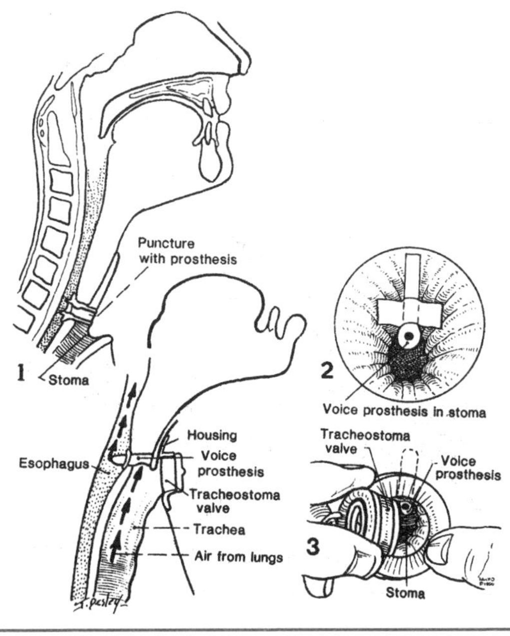

Note. From *Looking Forward: A Guidebook for the Laryngectomee* (3rd ed., p. 23), by R.L. Keith, 1995, New York: Thieme New York. Copyright 1995 by Thieme New York. Reprinted with permission.

in a permanent alteration in both function and appearance. Dysfunction relates to the sensorimotor deficits, such as changes in speech and swallowing. Changes in both function and appearance result in a process known as body image alteration, which often is accompanied by anxiety and depression (Dropkin, 1997). The process of coping with the dysfunction and disfigurement is referred to as body image reintegration and involves confronting the physical defects through resocialization and incorporating self-care activities into the daily routine (Dropkin, 1997). Nurses are very influential in assisting and teaching patients to cope with these changes (Sievers, 1997), and they must be sensitive and deliver care in a nonjudgmental and caring manner (Lockhart, 1999).

Effective coping strategies mediate the stress associated with head and neck cancer surgery (Dropkin, 2001). Preoperative assistance with coping, particularly with older patients, facilitates postoperative coping, with a possible reduction in length of hospital stay. Long-term follow-up aimed at monitoring posthospitalization coping effectiveness mediates stress on a continuous basis, thereby enhancing recovery and quality of life (Dropkin, 2001).

Conclusion

In *The Washington Post Magazine*, food and wine critic Donald Dresden (1978) explained his experience with laryngeal cancer. His brief but significant encounter with overcoming a handicap underscored the importance of determination. "Not everyone can return to the life he had before, but thousands do. It's more difficult to tell anyone now, but the champagne of life is sweeter after a brush with cancer of the larynx" (p. 46).

One of the major goals of cancer therapy is to preserve organs and organ function. It is hoped that the use of gene therapy will one day obviate the need for ablative head and neck surgery, thereby preserving the patient's self image. Cancer researchers have envied the selectivity of viruses for years: If they could only target cancer therapies to cancer cells and avoid damaging normal cells, they may be able to eliminate many of the noxious side effects of cancer treatment (Nettelbeck & Curiel, 2003). With less ablative surgery and the appropriate use of oncologic therapies, the sense organs, smell, sight, hearing, and voice will be preserved, offering the patient with head and neck cancer a more acceptable quality of life.

References

American Geriatrics Society. (1998). The management of chronic pain in older persons: AGS Panel on Chronic Pain in Older Persons. *Journal of the American Geriatrics Society, 46,* 635–651.

American Pain Society. (1995). Quality improvement guidelines for the treatment of acute pain and cancer pain: American Pain Society Quality of Care Committee. *JAMA, 274,* 1874–1880.

American Pain Society. (1999). *Principles of analgesic use in the treatment of acute pain and cancer pain* (4th ed.). Skokie, IL: Author.

Andresen, H.G., Cyr, M.H., Guadagnini, J., Hickey, M.M., Higgins, T.S., Huntoon, M.B., et al. (1998). General history, risk factors, and normal physical assessment. In L.L. Harris & M.B. Huntoon (Eds.), *Core curriculum for otorhinolaryngology and head-neck nursing* (pp. 9–32). New Smyrna Beach, FL: Society of Otorhinolaryngology and Head-Neck Nurses.

Arbogast, D. (2002). Enteral feedings with comfort and safety. *Clinical Journal of Oncology Nursing, 6,* 275–280.

ASPEN Board of Directors & The Clinical Guidelines Task Force. (2002). Guidelines for the use of parenteral and enteral nutrition in adult and pediatric patients. *Journal of Parenteral and Enteral Nutrition, 26*(Suppl. 1), 1SA–138SA.

Bockus, S. (1991). Troubleshooting your tube feedings. *American Journal of Nursing, 91*(5), 24–28.

Cheever, K.H. (1999). Early enteral feeding of patients with multiple trauma. *Critical Care Nurse, 19*(6), 40–51.

Cherny, N.I. (2000). The management of cancer pain. *CA: A Cancer Journal for Clinicians, 50,* 70–116.

Clarke, L.K. (1998). Rehabilitation for the head and neck cancer patient. *Oncology, 12,* 81–90.

Cutright, L.H., & Guadagnini, J.P. (1998). Oropharynx conditions and care. In L.L. Harris & M.B. Huntoon (Eds.), *Core curriculum for otorhinolaryngology and head-neck nursing* (pp. 207–226). New Smyrna Beach, FL: Society of Otorhinolaryngology and Head-Neck Nurses.

Devine, J.C., Potter, L.A., Magennis, P., Brown, J.S., & Vaughan, E.D. (2001). Flap monitoring after head and neck reconstruction: Evaluating an observation protocol. *Journal of Wound Care, 10,* 525–529.

Dresden, D. (1978, November 26). Speechless. *The Washington Post Magazine,* pp. 46–52.

Dropkin, M.J. (1989). Coping with disfigurement and dysfunction after head and neck surgery: A conceptual framework. *Seminars in Oncology Nursing, 5,* 213–219.

Dropkin, M.J. (1997). Postoperative body image in head and neck cancer patients. *Quality of Life: A Nursing Challenge, 5*(4), 110–114.

Dropkin, M.J. (2001). Anxiety, coping strategies, and coping behaviors in patients undergoing head and neck cancer surgery. *Cancer Nursing, 24,* 143–148.

Feldt, K.S. (2000). The checklist of nonverbal pain indicators (CNPI). *Pain Management Nursing, 1,* 13–21.

Folstein, M.F., Folstein, S.E., & McHugh, P.R. (1975). "Mini-mental state": A practical method for grading the cognitive state of patients for the clinician. *Journal of Psychiatric Research, 12*(3), 189–198.

Fuller, G. (1993). *Neurological examination made easy.* New York: Churchill Livingstone.

Goodrich, S.J., & Walker, A.I. (1997). Clinical swallow evaluation. In R. Leonard & K. Kendall (Eds.), *Dysphagia assessment and treatment planning: A team approach* (pp. 59–73). San Diego, CA: Singular.

Hahn, M.J., & Jones, A. (2000). *Head and neck nursing.* New York: Churchill Livingstone.

Harris, L.L. (1998). Patient problems. In L.L. Harris & M.B. Huntoon (Eds.), *Core curriculum for otorhinolaryngology and head-neck nursing* (pp. 309–325). New Smyrna Beach, FL: Society of Otorhinolaryngology and Head-Neck Nurses.

Hudak, M., & Bond-Domb, A. (1996). Postoperative head and neck cancer patients with artificial airways: The effects of saline lavage on tracheal mucus evacuation and oxygen saturation. *ORL—Head and Neck Nursing, 14*(1), 17–22.

Kendall, K.A., McKenzie, S.W., Leonard, R.J., & Jones, C. (1998). Structural mobility in deglutition after single modality treatment of head and neck carcinomas with radiotherapy. *Head and Neck, 20,* 720–725.

Kirsch, I., Jungeblut, A., Jenkins, L., & Kolstad, A. (1993). *Adult literacy in America: A first look at the results of the National Adult Literacy Survey* (2nd ed.). Washington, DC: Office of Educational Research and Improvement, U.S. Department of Education.

Krioukov, L.F. (1998). Principles for professional nursing practice. In L.L. Harris & M.B. Huntoon (Eds.), *Core curriculum for otorhinolaryngology and head-neck nursing* (pp. 1–5). New Smyrna Beach, FL: Society of Otorhinolaryngology and Head-Neck Nurses.

Ladage, E. (2003). Refeeding syndrome. *ORL—Head and Neck Nursing, 21*(3), 18–20.

Lockhart, J.S. (1999). Nurses' perceptions of head and neck oncology patients after surgery: Severity of facial disfigurement and patient gender. *ORL—Head and Neck Nursing, 17*(4), 12–25.

Logemann, J.A. (1997). *Evaluation and treatment of swallowing disorders* (2nd ed.). Austin, TX: Pro-Ed.

Maloney, J.P., Halbower, A.C., Fouty, B.F., Fagan, K.A., Balasubramaniam, V., Pike, A.W., et al. (2000). Systemic absorption of food dye in patients with sepsis. *New England Journal of Medicine, 343,* 1047–1048.

McCray, S., & Parrish, C.R. (2004). When chyle leaks: Nutrition management options. *Practical Gastroenterology, 28*(5), 60–76.

McKenzie, S. (1997). Swallow evaluation with videofluoroscopy. In R. Leonard & K. Kendall (Eds.), *Dysphagia assessment and treatment planning: A team approach* (pp. 83–101). San Diego, CA: Singular.

Metheny, N.A. (2002). Risk factors for aspiration. *Journal of Parenteral and Enteral Nutrition, 26*(Suppl. 6), S26–S33.

Metheny, N.A., Aud, M.A., & Wunderlich, R.J. (1999). A survey of bedside methods used to detect pulmonary aspiration of enteral formula in intubated tube-fed patients. *American Journal of Critical Care, 8,* 160–169.

Meyers, F.J., & Linder, J. (2003). Simultaneous care: Disease treatment and palliative care throughout illness. *Journal of Clinical Oncology, 21,* 1412–1415.

Miaskowski, C., Crews, J., Ready, L.B., Paul, S.M., & Ginsberg, B. (1999). Anesthesia-based pain services improve the quality of postoperative pain management. *Pain, 80,* 23–29.

Munro, C.L., & Grap, M.J. (2004). Oral health and care in the intensive care unit: State of the science. *American Journal of Critical Care, 13,* 25–33.

Nettelbeck, D., & Curiel, D. (2003). Tumor-busting viruses. *Scientific American, 289*(4), 68–75.

Patt, R.B. (1990). Non-pharmacologic measures for controlling oncologic pain. *American Journal of Hospice and Palliative Care, 7*(6), 30–37.

Pereira, J., & Phan, T. (2004). Management of bleeding in patients with advanced cancer. *Oncologist, 9,* 561–570.

Pujade-Lauraine, E., & Gascon, P. (2004). The burden of anemia in patients with cancer. *Oncology, 67*(Suppl. 1), 1–4.

Raymond, S.J. (1995). Normal saline instillation before suctioning: Helpful or harmful? A review of the literature. *American Journal of Critical Care, 4,* 267–271.

Schiech, L. (2000). Carotid artery rupture. *Clinical Journal of Oncology Nursing, 4,* 93–94.

Schwartz, S.L., & Barr, N.J. (1979). Carotid catastrophe. *American Journal of Nursing, 79,* 1566–1567.

Scolapio, J.S. (2002). Methods for decreasing risk of aspiration pneumonia in critically ill patients. *Journal of Parenteral and Enteral Nutrition, 26*(Suppl. 6), S58–S61.

Sievers, A.E.F. (1984). Nursing aspects. In P.J. Donald (Ed.), *Head and neck cancer: Management of the difficult case* (pp. 395–411). Philadelphia: W.B. Saunders.

Sievers, A.E.F. (1997). Nursing evaluation and care of the dysphagic patient. In R. Leonard & K. Kendall (Eds.), *Dysphagia assessment and treatment planning: A team approach* (pp. 41–59). San Diego, CA: Singular.

Sievers, A.E.F., & Donald, P.J. (1987). The use of bolus normal saline instillations in artificial airways: Is it useful or necessary? *Heart and Lung, 16,* 342–343.

Sigler, B.A. (1988). Nursing care of the head and neck cancer patient. *Oncology, 2*(12), 49–53.

Sigler, B.A., & Schuring, L. (1993). *Ear, nose, and throat disorders.* St. Louis, MO: Mosby.

Stannard, D., Puntillo, K., Miaskowski, C., Gleeson, S., Kehrle, K., & Nye, P. (1996). Clinical judgment and management of postoperative pain in critical care patients. *American Journal of Critical Care, 5,* 433–441.

Steele, S.R., Martin, M.J., Mullenix, P.S., Crawford, J.V., Cuadrado, D.S., & Andersen, C.A. (2004). Focused high-risk population screening for carotid arterial stenosis after radiation therapy for head and neck cancer. *American Journal of Surgery, 187,* 594–598.

Sykes, J., Johnson, R., & Hanks, G.W. (1997). ABC of palliative care. Difficult pain problems. *BMJ, 315,* 867–869.

Tamburri, L.M. (2000). Care of the patient with a tracheotomy. *Orthopaedic Nursing, 19*(2), 49–60.

van Bokhorst-de van der Schueren, M.A.E., Langendoen, S.I., Vondeling, H., Kuik, D., Quak, J.J., & van Leeuwen, P.A.M. (2000). Perioperative enteral nutrition and quality of life of severely malnourished head and neck cancer patients: A randomized clinical trial. *Clinical Nutrition, 19,* 437–444.

van Bokhorst-de van der Schueren, M.A.E., van Leeuwen, P.A., Kuik, D.J., Klop, W.M., Sauerwein, H.P., Snow, G.B., et al. (1999). The impact of nutritional status on the prognoses of patients with advanced head and neck cancer. *Cancer, 86,* 519–527.

Wiechula, R. (2003). The use of moist wound-healing dressings in the management of split-thickness skin graft donor sites: A systematic review. *International Journal of Nursing Practice, 9*(2), S9–S17.

World Health Organization. (1996). *Cancer pain relief with a guide to opioids availability* (2nd ed.). Geneva, Switzerland: Author.

CHAPTER 10

Survivorship

Penelope Stevens Fisher, MS, RN, CORLN

*There is no profit in curing the body, if in the process
we destroy the soul.*

Inscription on the Gate
City of Hope National Medical Center
Duarte, California

Introduction

Cancer survivorship begins when the person receiving the diagnosis hears what was told and reaches out for information, a treatment plan, and hope. The National Coalition for Cancer Survivorship (2004) defines a cancer survivor as "any individual that has been diagnosed with cancer, from the time of discovery and for the balance of life." An estimated 9.6 million survivors of cancer in the United States were alive in January 2000, and the overall five-year survival rate is 64% (American Cancer Society, 2005). This survival rate varies by the site, size, cell type, stage of cancer, and the time interval from detection to the start of treatment.

At the milestone of completing cancer treatment, the survivor once again faces untravelled ground and unknown expectations. The process and work of survivorship outcomes require expanded knowledge and roles for the oncology nurse and increased research to support intervention. Many survivors experience psychosociophysiologic and financial challenges, treatment effects, and lengthy rehabilitation. The loss of speech and learning a new method of communicating can be costly as well as cause an alteration in lifestyle. Disfigurement related to anatomic changes after surgical procedures may lead to coping issues and result in avoidance of social activities. For others, efforts must focus on maintaining quality of life during palliative care.

Prior to the 1990s, little nursing literature used the term *survivorship* as it related to cancer care. That body of knowledge has significantly increased. The National Cancer Policy Board and Institute of Medicine commissioned Ferrell, Virani, Smith, and Juarez (2003) to examine the role of oncology nurses in caring for the cancer survivor. The outcome was a review of existing oncology nursing standards, textbooks, research-based articles, nursing education, certification, and professional organizations that addressed issues of the cancer survivor, the caregiver, and the nurse. The data gathered from this work set a framework for the future (see Figure 10-1).

Figure 10-1. Role of Oncology Nurses in Survivorship

Conclusions and Recommendations: Role of Oncology Nursing to Ensure Quality Care for Cancer Survivors
1. Increase the focus by the Oncology Nursing Society (ONS) and other professional nursing groups on survivors and survivor issues.
2. Increase support for oncology specialty education within graduate programs, including the full spectrum of the cancer experience.
3. Evaluate and support oncology content in curricula, with emphasis on survivorship, which has received minimal attention in general oncology graduate programs.
4. Promote certification in oncology nursing through the OCN® and AOCN® examination process.
5. Explore opportunities to integrate survivorship content in basic nursing education (baccalaureate and associate degree) programs.
6. Increase support for oncology nursing research in survivorship, including
   • Support for expanded pilot funding through the National Institute of Nursing Research, ONS, and the ONS Foundation
   • Targeted research for areas not addressed in current research.
7. Support extensive continuing education for clinical nurses regarding survivorship because of the limited exposure in this area of undergraduate education.
8. Explore opportunities for nursing research in cancer survivorship in conjunction with clinical trials and cooperative groups.

Note. From "The Role of Oncology Nursing to Ensure Quality Care for Cancer Survivors: A Report Commissioned by the National Cancer Policy Board and Institute of Medicine," by B.R. Ferrell, R. Virani, S. Smith, and G. Juarez, 2003, *Oncology Nursing Forum, 30.* Retrieved March 16, 2005, from http://www.ons.org/publications/journals/ONF/Volume30/Issue1/300132.asp. Copyright 2003 by the Oncology Nursing Society. Reprinted with permission.

To understand the evolution of the current state of care for the cancer survivor, a look at early survivorship concepts is helpful. Leigh (1992) related survivorship to a model of time intervals and identified three stages: acute, extended, and permanent. During each stage, Leigh identified needs and applied the nursing process for care. Her work in 1998 further developed the model of time and increased the understanding of patients' psychosocial needs. In 2001, Leigh described the culture of cancer survivorship (see Table 10-1).

Previous chapters in this book describe the management of patient care during treatment of the primary head and neck cancer. During survivorship, this management continues; however, the foci may change. The survivor faces issues of determining the meaning of and obtaining and keeping quality of life. The survivor's perceptions of quality of life and the process to maintain it have been aided by family and friends, healthcare providers, and self-determination (Mellon, 2002). Oncology nurses have been paramount in identifying and defining the issues of cancer survivorship. Concerns include physiologic and psychosocial changes, late effects of treatment, short- and long-term complications, rehabilitation, fear of recurrence, economic burdens, spiritual effects, and palliative and end-of-life decisions (Dow, Ferrell, Haberman, & Eaton, 1999; Ganz, 2001; Leigh, 1992, 1998, 2001; O'Connor, Wicker, & Germino, 1990; Rowland, Aziz, Tesauro, & Fever, 2001; Zebrack, 2000, 2002).

Mellon (2002) explored the effects of cancer survivorship on family members. Finding positive meaning during survivorship helped to increase quality of life for survivors and families. Fear of recurrence became a chronic stressor but was lessened with genetic histories, early detection by monitoring exams, and expedient symptom management. Findings also suggested that existing strengths and styles of family communication could alter negative meaning and enhance quality of life. Nursing assessment in identification of these effects was critical to intervention for the process of survivorship.

Aziz and Rowland (2002) studied differences in cancer survivorship among ethnic minorities and the medically underserved. The American Cancer Society has reported survival rate statistics for minorities since 1974. Trends continue to define ethnic groups as having lower overall survival rates than Caucasian Americans. The authors noted that ethnic groups demonstrated issues related to past experiences, social mores, and cultural beliefs. These issues may affect coping, health behaviors, and use of resources differently than Caucasian American survivors. Education, access to care, and resources may be economically unavailable and/or the educational process nonexistent. Higher risks for second cancers may result from poorer health or behaviors that increase risk for cancer.

Cancer recurrences and second primaries, unfortunately, are not uncommon. The survivor lives with this fear daily (Leigh, 1998). When conventional therapy has not controlled the cancer, end-of-life decisions must be considered. Different approaches for care, comfort, and understanding are necessary to provide supportive care. Supportive care encompasses many meanings. When applied to curative therapy, it may be interpreted as care to augment the existing prescribed therapy. When used in the domain of palliative care, it is described as care to promote comfort without prolonging or hastening death (Prochoda & Seligman, 1997).

Survival Rates

Cancers of the head and neck remain as some of the most feared diseases. The cancer, treatment sequelae, and limitations of rehabilitation may significantly alter the survivor's lifestyle. Changes in body image, breathing, swallowing, and communicating may become disabilities. Rehabilitation and management of the changes may present many challenges to the survivor and the family. In addition to these obstacles, the patient faces survival statistics that can create continued fear of recurrence and death. Head and neck cancer survival rates are less than the overall average of 63% (see Table 10-2).

Rehabilitation

In the textbook *Essentials of Head and Neck Oncology* (Close, Larson, & Shah, 1998), several chapters discuss the

Table 10-1. The Culture of Cancer Survivorship				
Stage	Time Frame	Facing/Coping	Needs	Culture
Acute	Diagnosis through care	Fear, losses Acute side effects of therapy	Acute care Management Education	Erroneous information, myths Language barriers
Extended	End of initial treatment	Adjusting to compromises	Rehabilitation Support	Lack of understanding
Permanent	Remission Potentially cured	Adaptation Long-term/late effects of therapy	Insurance/financial security; managing late effects of treatment	Conflicting attitudes, beliefs, values
Note. Based on information from Leigh, 2001.				

Table 10-2. Head and Neck Cancer Relative Five-Year Survival Rates				
Site	All Stages %	Local %	Regional %	Distant %
Hypopharynx	35–40	–	–	–
Larynx	64.7	82.6	47.9	20.0
Oral cavity	58.7	81.0	50.7	29.5
Thyroid	95.8	99.3	95.5	59.9
Note. Based on information from American Cancer Society, 2005; Gray & O'Malley, 2001.				

analysis of rehabilitation. Rehabilitation is categorized as functional, prosthetic, and psychosocial. Functional rehabilitation focuses on speech, swallowing, shoulder motion, and facial nerve activity. Prosthetic rehabilitation provides devices to assist with oral cavity defects (obturators) or cosmesis (nose, eye, and ear prostheses). Psychosocial rehabilitation deals with coping mechanisms to adjust to physical and functional changes that may alter the survivor's lifestyle. Each of these types of rehabilitation presents opportunities for oncology nurses and a multidisciplinary and highly specialized care team. Research studies continue to explore the impact of cancer treatment on the survivor in regard to depression, pain, difficulties with social functioning and role, swallowing, speech, dry mouth, body image, presence of indwelling body tubes, shoulder function, substance abuse, and nutrition (Clarke, 1998; Dropkin, 1999; Fritz, 2001; Hanna et al., 2004; Pytynia et al., 2004; Taylor et al., 2004; Terrell et al., 2004).

Other characteristics of head and neck cancer survival have been studied. In the Terrell et al. (2004) study, survivors of head and neck cancer listed the presence of a feeding tube, medical comorbidities, the presence of a trachesotomy tube, chemotherapy, and neck dissections as predictors for quality of life. In this study, the two highest predictors were comorbidities and a feeding tube. Taylor et al. (2004) found that survivors who had undergone chemotherapy alone were 3.5 times more likely to have disabilities than those who did not receive chemotherapy. Those undergoing neck dissections had twice the chance of disability compared to survivors who did not have a neck dissection. Pain increased the odds of disability by 20%. Radiation therapy effects matched the disabilities of stage III or IV disease. However, disabilities decrease by 10% each decade of survival.

Costs

The cost of quality cancer care also may require that the survivor reestablish economic stability and, therefore, undergo financial rehabilitation. Brown, Riley, Schussler, and Etzioni (2002) used SEER-Medicare data to estimate cancer costs. Using the value of a dollar in 1996, head and neck cancer cost $1.6 billion. The cost included expenses for diagnostic testing,

hospitalization for surgery and chemotherapy, and standard radiation treatment. This equated to 4% of all cancer costs. The average Medicare payment per individual with head and neck cancer was $14,788. Head and neck cancer was listed as one of the 13 most common cancers, and 3.3% of all cancer costs were spent on patients with new head and neck cancers.

The cost of treatment correlates to the location, stage, and treatment modalities for the specific cancer. Cost of survivorship relates to the management of treatment side effects and rehabilitation of disabilities. This economic burden can be measured in direct and indirect costs (Terrell & Wilkins, 1998). Direct costs include monies needed for institutional and professional fees, medications, and durable medical equipment. Lang, Menzin, Earle, Jacobson, and Hsu (2004) used 1991–1993 SEER data to evaluate Medicare expenditures for older beneficiaries having newly diagnosed squamous cell cancer of the head and neck. A retrospective analysis of Medicare costs for initial treatments consisting of surgery and/or radiation and some chemotherapy was compared to a control group with no such diagnosis. The monies were converted to 1998 dollars, and the study found that Medicare payments would be three times higher than the control group payments. Statistics for advanced squamous cell cancer demonstrated higher costs as well. This suggested that the financial burden for squamous cell cancer of the head and neck may be higher than for other tumors.

Insurance

Health insurance is important to all cancer survivors. DeNavas-Walt, Proctor, and Mills (2004) reported that in 2003, an estimated 45 million people, or 15.6% of the population, did not have health insurance. Government-covered health insurance programs Medicaid and Medicare insured 35.6 million people (12.4%) and 39.5 million people (13.7%), respectively.

For the survivor of head and neck cancer engaged in functional, prosthetic, psychosocial, and economic rehabilitation, understanding and dealing with insurance policies, inquiries, and disclosures may become overwhelming. To offset company costs, insurance providers may discriminate against the survivors by raising premiums or may set time intervals before covering medical expenses. Insurance and care case managers, financial counselors, and advocacy groups may provide assistance (see Table 10-3).

Table 10-3. Community Economic Rehabilitation Resources (Limited List)

Resource	Contact Information
Financial	
CancerCare, Inc.	www.cancercare.org 800-813-4673
National Foundation for Credit Counseling	www.nfcc.org 800-388-2227
National Cancer Institute cancer information	www.cancer.gov 800-422-6237
OncoLink	www.oncolink.org
Pharmaceutical Research and Manufacturers of America—drug assistance	www.phrma.org 202-835-3400
Insurance	
American Cancer Society—insurance explanations	www.cancer.org 800-ACS-2345
America's Health Insurance Plans	www.ahip.org 202-778-3200
National Council on the Aging	www.ncoa.org 202-479-1200

Employment

Leigh and Thaler-DeMers (1997) found that 25% of cancer survivors experienced various types of employment discrimination. Methods of discrimination were identified as not being hired; being selected for a layoff; demotion; duty changes; failure to receive promotions or financial merit raises; and being perceived as unproductive workers. Taylor et al. (2004) found that 52% of the survivors of head and neck cancer studied were unable to return to work because of cancer treatment disabilities. Laws exist to prevent this type of discrimination, and advocacy groups continue to support this protection (see Table 10-4).

Support Groups

Support systems throughout the continuum of the head and neck cancer journey provide added opportunities for the survivor, family, and nursing staff. Building networks with others in the same situations creates new strengths for coping strategies and sets ideas about benchmarking for positive outcomes. Being able to talk to another about the similarities and differences of the individual's case helps to reinforce self-confidence and motivation.

Klemm and Hardie (2002) studied a common concern in survivorship—depression. They compared the traditional face-to-face support group method to the use of an Internet support group (contemporary). Previous literature supported

Table 10-4. Community Legal Rights and Advocacy Groups (Limited List)

Law	Purpose	Details
Consolidated Omnibus Budget Reconciliation Act (COBRA), 1986	Continues insurance	Must request within 60 days of leaving workplace
Health Insurance Portability and Accountability Act (HIPAA), 1996	Ensures insurance portability and accountability	Protects from denial of insurance based on preexisting health problems and sets guidelines for waiting period of coverage when changing employer group insurance
Family and Medical Leave Act (FMLA), 1993	Allows family and medical leaves	Provides up to 12 weeks of job-protected leave
Americans with Disabilities Act (ADA), 1990	Protects Americans with disabilities	Helps to prevent discrimination for disabilities and provides accommodations

Advocacy Resource	Contact Information
American Cancer Society	www.cancer.org 800-ACS-2345
National Coalition for Cancer Survivorship	www.canceradvocacy.org 877-622-7937
Patient Advocate Foundation	www.patientadvocate.org 800-532-5274

the value and success of the face-to-face method, but little research existed regarding outcomes of Internet support groups. A reliable and validated depression scale was used. Although variables existed among the participants, such as demographics, treatment phase, and beliefs about terminal status, only the treatment phase was significant to the level of depression. The Internet group had significantly higher depression scores than the face-to-face support group participants. The generation now surviving cancer is more Internet savvy and comfortable using the Internet as a resource.

This may require considerable rethinking for the oncology nurse in assessment and delivery of interventions for support. Nurses are instrumental in establishing support groups. The teaching and coordination skills of nurses promote partnering of survivors, other healthcare providers, social services, and community leaders to pool resources for support group development. Table 10-5 lists Internet and community resources for survivor support.

Table 10-5. Support Resources for Survivors of Head and Neck Cancer	
Support Resource	**Contact Information**
American Cancer Society	www.cancer.org 800-ACS-2345
American Academy of Otolaryngology—Head and Neck Surgery	www.entnet.org 703-836-4444
Cancer Survivors Online	www.cancersurvivors.org
Coalition of National Cancer Cooperative Groups CancerQuilt	www.cancertrialshelp.org/cancerQuilt
International Association of Laryngectomees	www.larynxlink.com
Let's Face It—Resources for patients with facial differences	www.faceit.org 360-676-7325
Oncology Nursing Society	www.ons.org 866-257-4667
Oncology Nursing Society's resource on cancer symptoms	www.cancersymptoms.org
Society of Otorhinolaryngology and Head-Neck Nurses, Inc.	www.sohnnurse.com 386-428-1695
Support for People with Oral and Head and Neck Cancer	www.spohnc.org 800-377-0928
Tobacco information and support links	www.tobacco.org
WebWhispers—Support for laryngectomees	www.webwhispers.org
Yul Brynner Head and Neck Cancer Foundation	www.headandneck.org 843-792-6624

Palliative Care

Recurrence and/or second primaries are common in cancer of the head and neck. The recurrence rate is 25%–28%, and the risk of a second primary per year is 3%–7% (Stack & Weymuller, 1998). Additionally, some stage III and IV cancers are incurable at the time of presentation. For these patients, the best supportive care may be palliative symptom management and assistance with end-of-life decisions.

The survivor is once again thrown into decisional conflict while reclarifying values, seeking possible additional treatment options, or coping with unpleasant symptoms of disease progression. The fear of recurrence becomes a reality, and the survivor once again must find strength to withstand the reevaluation of the situation, a new plan, and an amended outcome. Most likely, the psychosocial and physiologic changes will require additional care strategies.

In the patient with head and neck cancer, symptoms that require treatment are anorexia, dysphagia, airway management, and pain (Stack & Weymuller, 1998). Comfort and safety measures often must be creative and intense. Invasive tumors may cause wounds that are challenging because of bleeding, odor, or infection. McMillan and Weitzner (2000) found that dyspnea and constipation were, in addition to pain, the most troubling symptoms in patients receiving hospice care. The combination of these symptoms may cause the acuity of care to become too burdensome for the family. Patients and families therefore may need assistance in the home to manage care. Home health agencies and hospices have become invaluable in supervising care, providing durable medical equipment, and coordinating the multidisciplinary team to meet the needs of the patient.

Additionally, support systems for family and patient, such as volunteer sitters, shopper services, housekeeping, transportation, and grief and bereavement counseling, are available through most hospice agencies. Some hospices have inpatient facilities that offer respite services.

Reb (2003) published a comprehensive policy analysis on palliative and end-of-life care. The study reviewed multiple care settings, legislative protection and activities, quality standards, costs, nursing roles, and education. The author concluded that integrating palliative care throughout the course of illness could provide improved symptom management, quality of life, and continuity of care along with referrals to hospices in a more timely manner. Resources for palliative care and end-of-life decisions are listed in Table 10-6.

Summary

Throughout this book, nursing care has been addressed. When relating it to a survivor of head and neck cancer, it seems appropriate to correlate nursing care with Leigh's (1992) model. The acute stage of survivorship is the assess-

Table 10-6. Resources for Palliative Care and End-of-Life Decisions	
Organization	**Web Site**
Center to Advance Palliative Care	www.capcmssm.org
International Association for Hospice and Palliative Care	www.hospicecare.com
National Hospice and Palliative Care Organization	www.nhpco.org

ment process. It is the proving ground for the novice of the disease to learn of his or her needs and abilities to understand what the challenge is. The nursing staff provides, directs, and demonstrates immediate care, which formulates the beginning of rehabilitation. The extended stage relates to the intermediate survivor who accepts the challenge to demand excellence in rehabilitation. The third stage, permanency, holds the expert strategist who has regained function and confidence and whose life is near normal. Maslow's concept of self-actualization (as cited in Volker, 1992) has returned. The survivor now can give back to others. Yet even with this gained self-confidence, the fear of cancer recurrence remains. To that end, the nurse remains the instiller of hope.

The nurse serves as the teacher, mentor, facilitator, validator, supporter, and evaluator and, with the rest of the team, coordinates the journey. Every tool and intervention known to nursing is used when and where required. At the completion of the task, whether it be a complete cure and recovery or the finality of death, the outcome is the same: One caring spirit who is there to help another to survive.

References

American Cancer Society. (2005). *Cancer facts and figures, 2005.* Atlanta, GA: Author.

Aziz, N.M., & Rowland, J.H. (2002). Cancer survivorship research among ethnic minority and medically underserved groups. *Oncology Nursing Forum, 29,* 789–801.

Brown, M.L., Riley, G.F., Schussler, N., & Etzioni, R.D. (2002). Estimating health care costs related to cancer treatment from SEER-Medicare data. *Medical Care, 40*(Suppl. 8), IV-104–117. Retrieved July 27, 2004, from http://progressreport.cancer.gov/doc.asp?pid=1&did=21&chid=13&coid=33&mid=vpco

Clarke, L.K. (1998). Rehabilitation for the head and neck cancer patient. *Oncology, 12,* 81–89.

Close, L.G., Larson, D.L., & Shah, J.P. (Eds.). (1998). *Essentials of head and neck oncology.* New York: Thieme.

DeNavas-Walt, C., Proctor, B.D., & Mills, R.J. (2004, August). *Income, poverty, and health insurance coverage in the United States: 2003.* Washington, DC: U.S. Government Printing Office. Retrieved March 23, 2004, from http://www.census.gov/prod/2004pubs/p60-226.pdf

Dow, K.H., Ferrell, B.R., Haberman, M.R., & Eaton, L. (1999). The meaning of quality of life in cancer survivorship. *Oncology Nursing Forum, 26,* 519–528.

Dropkin, M.J. (1999). Body image and quality of life after head and neck cancer surgery. *Cancer Practice, 7,* 309–313.

Ferrell, B.R., Virani, R., Smith, S., & Juarez, G. (2003). The role of oncology nursing to ensure quality care for cancer survivors: A report commissioned by the National Cancer Policy Board and Institute of Medicine. *Oncology Nursing Forum, 30,* E1–E11. Retrieved March 16, 2005, from http://www.ons.org/publications/journals/ONF/Volume30/Issue1/300132.asp

Fritz, D.J. (2001). Life experiences of head and neck cancer survivors: A pilot study. *ORL—Head and Neck Nursing, 19*(4), 9–13.

Ganz, P.A. (2001). Late effects of cancer and its treatment. *Seminars in Oncology Nursing, 17,* 241–248.

Gray, W.C., & O'Malley, B.W. (2001). Neoplasms of the hypopharynx. In C.M. Alper, E.N. Myers, & D.E. Eibling (Eds.), *Decision making in ear, nose, and throat disorders* (pp. 176–177). Philadelphia: W.B. Saunders.

Hanna, E., Sherman, A., Cash, D., Adams, D., Vural, E., Fan, C.Y., et al. (2004). Quality of life for patients following total laryngectomy vs. chemoradiation for laryngeal preservation. *Archives of Otolaryngology—Head and Neck Surgery, 130,* 875–879.

Klemm, P., & Hardie, T. (2002). Depression in Internet and face-to-face cancer support groups: A pilot study. *Oncology Nursing Forum, 29,* 345–351.

Lang, K., Menzin, J., Earle, C.C., Jacobson, J., & Hsu, M.A. (2004). The economic cost of squamous cell cancer of the head and neck: Findings from linked SEER-Medicare data. *Archives of Otolaryngology—Head and Neck Surgery, 130,* 1269–1275.

Leigh, S. (1992). Cancer survivorship issues. In J.C. Clark & R.F. McGee (Eds.), *Core curriculum for oncology nursing* (2nd ed., pp. 257–262). Philadelphia: W.B. Saunders.

Leigh, S. (1998). Survivorship. In C.C. Burke (Ed.), *Psychosocial dimensions of oncology nursing care* (pp. 129–149). Pittsburgh, PA: Oncology Nursing Society.

Leigh, S. (2001). The culture of survivorship. *Seminars in Oncology Nursing, 17,* 234–235.

Leigh, S.A., & Thaler-DeMers, D. (1997). Survivorship. In R.A. Gates & R.M. Fink (Eds.), *Oncology nursing secrets* (pp. 411–418). Philadelphia: Hanley & Belfus.

McMillan, S.C., & Weitzner, M. (2000). How problematic are various aspects of quality of life in patients with cancer at end of life? *Oncology Nursing Forum, 27,* 817–824.

Mellon, S. (2002). Comparisons between cancer survivors and family members on meaning of the illness and family quality of life. *Oncology Nursing Forum, 29,* 1117–1125.

National Coalition for Cancer Survivorship. (2004). *Glossary.* Retrieved January 10, 2005, from http://www.canceradvocacy.org/resources/glossary.aspx#5

O'Connor, A.P., Wicker, C.A., & Germino, B.B. (1990). Understanding the cancer patient's search for meaning. *Cancer Nursing, 13,* 167–175.

Prochoda, K.P., & Seligman, P.A. (1997). Palliative care. In R.A. Gates & R.M. Fink (Eds.), *Oncology nursing secrets* (pp. 304–311). Philadelphia: Hanley & Belfus.

Pytynia, K.B., Grant, J.R., Etzel, C.J., Roberts, D., Wei, Q., & Sturgis, E.M. (2004). Matched analysis of survival in patients with squamous cell carcinoma of the head and neck diagnosed before and after 40 years of age. *Archives of Otolaryngology—Head and Neck Surgery, 130,* 869–873.

Reb, A. (2003). Palliative and end-of-life care: Policy analysis. *Oncology Nursing Forum, 30,* 35–50.

Rowland, J.H., Aziz, N., Tesauro, G., & Fever, E.J. (2001). The changing face of cancer survivorship. *Seminars in Oncology Nursing, 17,* 236–240.

Stack, B.C., & Weymuller, E.A. (1998). Supportive care. In L.G. Close, D.L. Larson, & J.P. Shah (Eds.), *Essentials of head and neck oncology* (pp. 416–424). New York: Thieme.

Taylor, J.C., Terrell, J.E., Ronis, D.L., Fowler, K.E., Bishop, C., Lambert, M.T., et al. (2004). Disability in patients with head and neck cancer. *Archives of Otolaryngology—Head and Neck Surgery, 130,* 764–769.

Terrell, J.E., Ronis, D.L., Fowler, K.E., Bradford, C.R., Chepeha, D.B., Prince, M.E., et al. (2004). Clinical predictors of quality of life in patients with head and neck cancer. *Archives of Otolaryngology—Head and Neck Surgery, 130,* 401–407.

Terrell, J.E., & Wilkins, E.G. (1998). Outcomes and cost effectiveness of contemporary head and neck treatment. In L.G. Close, D.L. Larson, & J.P. Shah (Eds.), *Essentials of head and neck oncology* (pp. 425–432). New York: Thieme.

Volker, D. (1992). Standards of oncology nursing practice. In J.C. Clark & R.F. McGee (Eds.), *Core curriculum for oncology nursing* (2nd ed., pp. 3–17). Philadelphia: W.B. Saunders.

Zebrack, B.J. (2000). Cancer survivors and quality of life: A critical review of the literature. *Oncology Nursing Forum, 27,* 1395–1401.

Zebrack, B.J. (2002). Cancer survivor identity and quality of life. *Cancer Practice, 8,* 238–242.

CHAPTER 11

Nursing Research Issues

Mary Jo Dropkin, PhD, RN

Introduction

According to the Oncology Nursing Society's (2004) position "Cancer Research and Cancer Clinical Trials," the goal of nursing research is to improve the lives of those who have been affected by cancer. The purpose of this chapter is to present an overview of clinical nursing research findings published within the past 25 years, to summarize the findings, and to identify future directions based on the current state of the science in head and neck cancer nursing. To that end, a literature search has been conducted using the Long Island University's Brooklyn Campus Library, Medline, CINAHL, and Dissertation Abstracts International. This chapter is organized according to the Recovery Model, as developed by Scott and Eisendrath (1986), to categorize the diverse clinical areas in which primary nursing studies have been conducted and to describe as well as synthesize the results. These areas include the physical, functional, cognitive, and emotional dimensions of recovery following diagnosis and treatment for head and neck cancer.

Physical Recovery: Surgical Treatment

According to the Recovery Model (Scott & Eisendrath, 1986), physical recovery is conceptualized as biophysiologic adjustment under the conditions of head and neck cancer, its treatment, and perceived stress associated with the illness. Manifestations of this include signs and symptoms of the disease, attribution of symptoms to the disease, and the sequelae of treatment. The manner in which the patient with head and neck cancer tolerates treatment or reduces sequelae through self-care constitutes the process of physical recovery (Scott & Eisendrath). Based on the literature reviewed, primary areas for study in patients with head and neck cancer undergoing surgery include biophysical compromises associated with the disease and surgical treatment, such as eating difficulties and postoperative facial disfigurement and associated dysfunc-

tions; factors that affect tolerance of surgical treatment, such as age, gender, and previous treatment; sequelae of surgical treatment, such as pain and gastrointestinal distress; and self-care. For those patients treated with radiation therapy (RT), the predominant physical recovery issues addressed were sequelae of treatment including pain, mucositis, and fatigue. Self-care designed to reduce these sequelae also was a focus of nursing study. Finally, the sequelae of stomatitis and altered eating strategies were the primary aims of research related to physical recovery from chemotherapy.

Biophysical Changes

Eating Difficulties

Langius, Bjorvell, and Lind (1993) noted eating disabilities in a sample of 29 patients both before (group 1, n = 13) and after presurgical RT (group 2, n = 16). The researchers used questionnaires to collect data. Eating disabilities were evident in both groups. Group 2, however, experienced a significant increase in eating problems, such as changes in taste and scent/smell, xerostomia, and difficulty chewing. Mouth pain also was reported by 54% of the patients in group 1 and 50% in group 2, primarily from the cancer site.

Disfigurement and Dysfunction

Visible facial disfigurement and impairment of local function(s) clearly represent the most emergent and dramatic physical changes related to surgical treatment for head and neck cancer. To measure the perception of severity of disfigurement and dysfunction following radical head and neck cancer surgery, Dropkin, Malgady, Scott, Oberst, and Strong (1983) developed a scale to quantify these concepts. The sample consisted of 100 female RNs employed at a large urban cancer center. Subjects judged the relative severity of disfigurement following 11 routinely performed surgical procedures as well as the eight attendant sensorimotor dysfunctions. Statistical analysis demonstrated that separate scales of severity exist for disfigurement and dysfunction following major head and neck cancer surgery. Judgments of the perceived severity of disfigurement were independent of the perceived severity of dysfunction. Three of the five most severely rated disfigurative procedures involved resection of the mandible and were clinically associated with permanent dysfunctions (impairment of speech and mastication). Perception of severity was not contingent upon the volume of tissue removed. Rather, the procedures considered to be most severely disfigurative involved major structural alteration in the center of the face, the region providing the greatest audiovisual stimuli in interaction with others. Additionally, three of the major sense organs are located in this region. Clinically, these findings indicated that disfigurement and dysfunction are two separate entities in the patient's recovery process. The high degree of agreement within the sample of RNs suggested that consensus exists on the impact of category of disfigurement and dysfunction upon the patient and the nurse, emphasizing the need to further address the possible influence of clinicians' perceptions on their interaction with patients.

Lockhart (2000) used a comparative descriptive design to determine differences of female nurses' perceptions regarding the severity of facial disfigurement in patients following head and neck cancer surgery. The sample consisted of two groups of female nurses, 30 experienced and 30 inexperienced in head and neck oncology. Subjects completed a Modified Disfigurement Scale adapted from Dropkin et al.'s (1983) Disfigurement/Dysfunction Scale. In contrast to previous findings, these results indicated that differences in nurses' perceptions of disfigurement were a function of patient gender but not significantly related to their experience. In support of previous research, however, the study determined that nurses perceived surgical procedures involving the central portion of the face as more disfiguring than those procedures involving the periphery of the face.

Tolerance Factors

Age

Kagan et al. (2002) conducted a study designed to determine the effect of patient age on postoperative pathway length of stay for complex head and neck surgical resections. The sample consisted of 43 patients. The study analyzed age, comorbid status, and postoperative complications in relation to impact on length of hospitalization. A prepathway group of 87 consecutive patients was used for comparison. Results of this study indicated that the average length of stay significantly increased by 25% for patients older than the age of 65. The findings supported a clinical association among advancing age, comorbidity, and surgical complications. However, age was not statistically associated with the occurrence of comorbidity, complications, or the combination of the two. The trends toward an association among length of stay, age, comorbidity, and complications, rather, are interpreted as a manifestation of declining functional reserve, a concept com-

mon in geriatric practice. Ultimately, these results supported that older adults tend to tolerate head and neck cancer surgery in a manner that is not significantly different from younger adults. The researchers concluded, however, that older age creates a clinically significant increase in resource utilization by virtue of increased length of hospital stay. These findings clarified the results of previous research findings that older subjects sustained more disfigurative surgery and ultimately experienced prolonged hospitalization (Dropkin, 1997).

Gender

In a study designed to examine factors contributing to the length of hospital stay (Dropkin, 1997), out of 117 adults about to undergo head and neck cancer surgery, gender (female) was significantly and positively related to hospital stay. The findings showed that women tended to stay longer than men. The researcher subsequently concluded that females about to undergo head and neck cancer surgery may be identified as "high risk" for extended hospitalization.

Previous Treatment

The same study (Dropkin, 1997) also determined that those participants who had undergone previous RT or chemotherapy prior to surgery similarly experienced extended length of postoperative hospitalization.

Postoperative Complications

Postoperative complications constituted the strongest predictor of length of hospitalization (Dropkin, 1997). These problems mainly consisted of wound healing complications, such as fistula formation. The actual number of complications was too small to submit to correlation or for regression analysis. It is interesting to note, however, that although preoperative RT and/or chemotherapy might be expected to contribute directly to variance in postoperative wound healing or infection problems with subsequent extension of hospitalization, these treatments emerged as independent predictors of variance in length of hospital stay. Forty percent (n = 46) of this sample underwent preoperative RT and/or chemotherapy, indicating that at the time of this study, surgical treatment and hospitalization were considered "last resort" measures in the face of treatment failure. The significant relationships between pretreatment and length of hospital stay suggested that the rigorous and relatively long-term preoperative treatment(s) of RT and/or chemotherapy significantly affected one's physical tolerance of surgical treatment.

Sequelae of Treatment

Pain

In a phenomenologic pilot study designed to describe the experiences of three patients (two males, one female) who survived head and neck cancer treatment, Fritz (2001) noted that two of the three participants identified neck and shoulder pain as a chronic problem since the time of their surgical treatment. One male participant felt that the pain was tolerable; the female, two years following surgery, felt the pain was increasing. The participant attributed this pain to possible recurrence. The third patient complained of an extremely stiff neck that he perceived to be very painful "even to touch."

Alterations in Eating

A study by Lennie, Christman, and Jadack (2001) was designed to describe altered patterns of eating and nutrition following total laryngectomy. A total of 36 participants were surveyed by mail. Results indicated that the greatest impact of the surgery on eating was the time required to eat a meal. Forty-two percent identified decreased overall enjoyment of eating related to postsurgical anosmia. Although a reduction in sense of taste was reported, the sample was not stratified according to treatment modality (i.e., adjuvant RT or chemotherapy in addition to total laryngectomy). Subsequently, patient difficulties such as increased time to eat may, in fact, be related to xerostomia, not the surgical procedure. The results of this study must be interpreted with extreme caution because of such methodologic errors. However, it represents an attempt to further investigate patients' adjustment to the specific biophysical compromises imposed by head and neck cancer surgery.

Gastrointestinal Distress

Reese et al. (1996) conducted a study to determine the difference in the incidence of diarrhea among subjects given one of three formulas with varying concentrations of fiber administered by nasogastric tube (NGT). The study also examined variables affecting incidence of diarrhea, discomfort other than diarrhea associated with NGT tube feedings, and effects of changing from continuous to interval feedings on incidence of diarrhea. In a prospective, double-blind design, 80 subjects undergoing head and neck cancer surgery that required an NGT tube postoperatively were randomly assigned to receive one of three formulas: isotonic fiber-free formula, isotonic 14 g fiber/l formula, or isotonic 7 g fiber/l formula. Patients who had experienced gastrointestinal illness within two weeks prior to surgery were excluded from study. Through the use of medical records as well as a preadmission interview, the researchers obtained information on subjects' dietary habits and food aversions, current medications, history of alcohol and tobacco use, and comorbid conditions. Subjects were monitored daily for rate and volume of formula administration, stool frequency and consistency, frequency of gastrointestinal discomfort such as heartburn, nausea, fullness, cramping, flatulence, and vomiting, as well as use of antibiotics and analgesics. The results of multiple logistic regression showed significant odds ratios for developing diarrhea in females, subjects who had prior food aversions, and subjects receiving broad-spectrum antibiotics. Diarrhea was four times more likely to occur in male subjects who had received a fiber-free formula. A total of 70% of the sample experienced gastrointestinal distress with continuous feedings, and 50% experienced discomforts when advanced to interval feedings. Researchers concluded that fiber formulas reduced the incidence of diarrhea in male, but not female, subjects. Moreover, the effect of antibiotics paralleled previous findings in the literature. Based on these results, the investigators included specific implications for practice, such as use of formulas with fiber for male patients. Although liquid stools do not warrant interruption of tube feeding, gastrointestinal discomforts do. Finally, interval feeding schedules require monitoring similar to continuous feeding schedules.

Self-Care

The Disfigurement/Dysfunction Scale (Dropkin et al., 1983) was used in a comprehensive descriptive study that examined the relationship between the degree of disfigurement/dysfunction and postoperative self-care (Dropkin & Scott, 1983). The theoretical framework underlying this study is the Stress-Coping Model (Scott, Oberst, & Dropkin, 1980). The sample consisted of 51 male and female patients who underwent radical head and neck cancer surgery. At that time, a major postoperative nursing recommendation included self-care, ostensibly basic tasks. Following major head and neck surgery, however, self-care implies close viewing or touching of the defect. Self-care was operationally defined as performance of (a) basic hygiene, (b) tasks specifically associated with the surgical procedure and taught by the nursing staff, and (c) grooming. Grooming was operationally defined as a self-care task motivated by the desire to improve appearance, such as shaving in men, makeup application in women, and hair arrangement for both. Grooming also requires the patient to look in a mirror or visually confront the head and neck defect. The time frame for study was postoperative days 4–6. Findings revealed significant negative relationships between severity of disfigurement and self-care tasks. These results implied that severity of disfigurement is related more to delay in the recovery process than dysfunction. This may be explained by the fact that dysfunction is less visually dramatic, often is temporary, and may be assisted by artificial means, improved through rehabilitation efforts, or totally regained. Dysfunction seems related to the ongoing manner in which the self has been presented throughout life rather than to sudden changes in facial appearance, criteria more dependent on social convention. It was concluded that, generally, postoperative days 4–6 can be considered to be a pivotal period in the recovery process in terms of acceptance of the defect. Significant increases in all head and neck tasks, regardless of difficulty level or need for visualization, occurred between postoperative days 4–5. Baker (1992) later disputed this sequence of recovery; however, the findings must be interpreted with extreme caution because of methodologic errors.

Physical Recovery: Radiation Therapy

According to the literature reviewed on physical recovery and RT in the patient population with head and neck cancer, primary areas for study included the biophysiologic compromises associated with RT-induced mucosal injury, oropharyngeal pain, mucositis-related pain, and xerostomia. Tolerance factors were related to additional treatment, such as surgery and/or chemotherapy, the primary cancer site, dental prophylaxis/oral treatment, and RT complications. Sequelae of treatment studied included weight loss, dysphonia, difficulty opening the mouth, taste changes, skin changes, lethargy, weakness, and sleep disturbance. Three studies examined self-care.

Biophysiologic Changes

Mucositis

The condition of RT-induced oral mucositis is not consistently defined among the studies reviewed. Mucositis was found to occur, however, across all samples under study. It has been subjectively described as "mouth sores . . . mouth pain and irritation" (Rose-Ped et al., 2002, p. 463). It also is observable (Huang, Wilkie, Schubert, & Ting, 2000) and measurable (Dodd et al., 2003; Shiba, 1997). It typically develops within approximately 2.5 weeks (Dodd et al.; Rose-Ped et al.) after initiation of treatment. According to Dodd et al.'s findings, severity of mucositis is not necessarily related to the RT dose received nor to pain on swallowing. From its onset, mucositis typically lasts throughout the course of treatment (Shiba) and may, in fact, persist for more than eight weeks after completion of treatment (Rose-Ped et al.).

Pain

In a symptom profile of patients receiving RT for nasopharyngeal cancer, Huang et al. (2000) noted complaints of oropharyngitis in a sample of 37 participants during weeks 3–7 of treatment. These results must be interpreted with some caution, however, because 46% of the sample had received chemotherapy prior to initiation of RT.

Because of the morbidity associated with RT to the head and neck region, Rose-Ped et al. (2002) designed an investigation to characterize the effects of RT from the patient's perspective. A total of 33 patients who had previously undergone RT with or without chemotherapy for the treatment of head and neck cancer were recruited from five metropolitan areas. The subjects participated in an in-depth interview about their experience. The interview consisted of open- and closed-ended questions. A limitation of the study is that patients' responses are based on their recollection of treatment that had occurred several years earlier. Length of time since treatment for the majority of the sample was five years (52%); one-third underwent treatment in 1996–1997 and 15% during or before 1995. Although participants recollected pain to be the overall worst part of the treatment experience, only 38% of the patients reported it on interview. Specifically, 20% reported pharyngitis-related pain and 18% mucositis-related pain as the most debilitating aspect of treatment.

In contrast, Shiba (1997) concluded that all participants in a sample of 49 individuals undergoing RT to the head and neck region developed oropharyngeal pain. Moreover, subjects in this sample reported that the pain increased in severity throughout the course of treatment. Significant differences in the level of pain occurred whether the patient was swallowing at all data collection points. Increasingly severe pain was reported on swallowing as early as week 2 of treatment. Similarly, pain on swallowing was reported by a subsample of 18 patients with head and neck cancer in a study by Ohrn and Sjoden (2003). In contrast, Dodd et al. (2003) found no significant differences in pain on swallowing in their sample of 30 patients with head and neck cancer undergoing RT. Participants were evaluated at the onset of mucositis (weeks 1–2 of treatment), at the end of treatment, and one month following completion of treatment.

Xerostomia

One study was designed to evaluate the effectiveness of vegetable oil for treatment of xerostomia (Walizer & Ephraim, 1996). The study also investigated the relationship between observed oral pathology and subjective reports of dryness. The sample consisted of 29 adults with head and neck cancer who were at least four weeks post-RT. Vegetable oil was compared with a standard artificial saliva product, Xerolube® (Colgate-Palmolive, New York, NY). At the time of entry into study, all patients were examined for oral pathology before being randomly assigned to an experimental or control group. Each subject served as his or her own control. Participants received two weeks of each treatment with a two-week "washout" period between therapies. Clinical evaluation for oral pathology, as well as subjective evaluation of dryness, was conducted every two weeks for a total of eight weeks. Findings suggested that both Xerolube and vegetable oil reduced dryness during RT. Although vegetable oil neither improved nor reduced oral health, it did diminish subjects' oral dryness.

In a qualitative analysis of survivors of head and neck cancer, Fritz (2001) described a patient's subjective experience of xerostomia. Similarly, Rose-Ped et al.'s (2002) participants noted the occurrence of "loss of saliva or dry mouth" (p. 463). Shiba (1997) reported severe xerostomia related to treatment that was distressing to the subjects. In the sample treated for nasopharyngeal primary cancer, xerostomia was reported as moderate to severe (Huang et al., 2000).

Tolerance Factors

Additional Treatment(s)

In the sample of patients undergoing RT for nasopharyngeal cancer, Huang et al. (2000) found a significant increase in severity of oropharyngeal pain and difficulty swallowing in those participants who had undergone previous chemotherapy. In Rose-Ped et al.'s (2002) sample, 42% of the population had undergone surgical treatment. Nearly half had received induction chemotherapy with the start of RT, with approximately 40% receiving concurrent chemotherapy and RT. Only 13% of this sample underwent RT prior to chemotherapy. Overall, about half (45%) received chemotherapy in addition to surgery and/or RT. Additional treatment(s) are not accounted for, however, in description of the nature or severity of symptoms or stress experienced. Subsequently, the results must be interpreted with some caution.

Primary Site

Participants in Rose-Ped et al.'s (2002) investigation had been diagnosed with tongue, mouth, tonsil, oropharynx, nasopharynx, hypopharynx, larynx, thyroid, and salivary gland primary head and neck cancer sites. Specific treatment modalities were contingent on the type of cancer as well as the geographic area where the patients received treatment. In some instances, primary site and subsequent RT predicted changes in the experience of treatment. For example, all participants with tongue cancer reported the sensation of changes in the oral cavity, whereas only 25% of the sample with a primary cancer located in the neck reported change in the condition of their mouths.

Dental Prophylaxis and Oral Treatment

Approximately 61% of Rose-Ped et al.'s (2002) sample had received an oral examination by a dentist or oral surgeon prior to initiation of RT. Sixty-five percent of those participants reported that oral care, such as a mouthwash or rinse, was usually prescribed. Dodd et al. (2003) conducted a pilot study to compare the effectiveness of micronized sucralfate (Carafate® [Axcan Scandipharm, Birmingham, AL]) mouthwash to salt and soda mouthwash in terms of severity of mucositis, mucositis-related pain, and healing time for RT-induced mucositis in a sample of 30 patients with head and neck cancer. No significant differences were determined in the number of days to onset of mucositis nor to pain ratings upon swallowing during treatment, at the end of treatment, or at the one-month follow-up assessment. Researchers concluded that, given no significant differences in efficacy between the micronized sucralfate and salt and soda, the use of salt and soda for oral care during RT would be more prudent as well as cost effective.

Radiation Therapy Complications

Of the studies reviewed, two reported participants requiring hospitalization as a result of RT complications. Rose-Ped et al.'s (2002) findings included that 27% of the sample were hospitalized because of treatment complications, such as dehydration, inability to eat or drink, mouth pain, extreme weakness, and fatigue. The mean length of hospital stay was 5.7 days with a range of 1–14 days. Twenty percent of Shiba's

(1997) sample required unscheduled hospitalization for treatment complications. An additional nine (18%) patients visited emergency rooms for such problems.

Sequelae of Treatment

Weight Loss

As a result of pain and burning in the oropharynx, patients diagnosed with a variety of primary sites may be unable to eat, drink, swallow, or experience taste changes (Rose-Ped et al., 2002; Shiba, 1997). In addition, all patients undergoing RT for cancer of the nasopharynx also experienced difficulty opening their mouths (Huang et al., 2000). Subsequently, severe weight loss often is associated with treatment. Eighty-three percent of Rose-Ped et al.'s sample reported substantial weight loss ranging from 12–79 pounds, with a mean weight loss of 29 pounds. Of these, 29% required gastric tube implantation.

Additional Sequelae

Twenty-nine percent of Rose-Ped et al.'s (2002) sample reported difficulty talking or dysphonia. The time frame during which this occurred, in relation to treatment, was not specified.

Two investigations (Rose-Ped et al., 2002; Shiba, 1997) identified taste changes ranging from complete loss of taste to reduced taste.

Huang et al. (2000) reported skin changes. In this sample, skin problems generally did not present until week 4 of treatment.

Weakness and fatigue were reported as cause for hospitalization in one study (Rose-Ped et al., 2002). In another study by Meek et al. (2000), designed to test the psychometric properties of several fatigue instruments for use with patients with cancer, a cohort of patients with head and neck cancer receiving RT was included in the sample. However, there was a 65% attrition rate in this group, all of whom were male. The reasons for this attrition were not addressed.

In Rose-Ped et al.'s (2002) sample, 25% reported sleep disturbance. The possible sources of sleep disturbance were not discussed.

Self-Care

Self-care was examined using Orem's Theory of Self-Care to explore the perceived need for change in universal and health-deviated self-care activity (Jaster, 1991). The sample consisted of 11 patients undergoing external beam RT for head and neck cancer and who had completed two-thirds of their treatment. Results indicated that coming for and receiving treatment as well as the need for a special diet were the most burdensome health-deviated activities. Of the universal self-care activities, working, eating, and performing household tasks or errands were most burdensome.

Shiba (1997) found that self-care activities only moderately relieved pain, mouth sores, and xerostomia, symptoms for which patients used the most self-care activities. Finally, self-care was inherent in participation in Dodd et al.'s (2003) study. All patients carried out a systematic oral hygiene protocol throughout the course of treatment.

Physical Recovery: Chemotherapy

According to the literature reviewed on physical recovery and chemotherapy in the patient population with head and neck cancer, the targeted areas for study included biophysiologic changes and sequelae of treatment.

Biophysiologic Changes

Forty-six percent of Huang et al.'s (2000) sample of participants (N = 37) had received chemotherapy prior to initiation of RT. The investigators concluded that sequential chemotherapy and RT were associated with significantly more severe oropharyngeal problems, including dry mouth, taste changes, difficulty swallowing, hoarseness, sore throat, and mucositis, than RT alone. No significant differences were found in other areas, such as skin problems.

Sequelae of Treatment

A cohort of 20 patients with head and neck cancer undergoing chemotherapy participated in the development of the Eating During Treatment Survey (EDTS), which was designed to measure symptom experience and eating strategies (Wilson, 1993). Content validity, construct validity, and internal consistency were adequately demonstrated. Although further testing is needed prior to use of this questionnaire in the clinical setting, it was concluded that the EDTS appears promising in that it may be used with patients with head and neck cancer to more clearly define the relationship between symptoms related to chemotherapy treatment and eating difficulties.

Summary: Physical Recovery

Patients' physical response to diagnosis and treatment for head and neck cancer constitutes the vast majority of the literature reviewed. Overall, 18 studies were reviewed, 9 of which primarily focused on patients undergoing surgical treatment; 8, RT; and 1, chemotherapy. Of the studies related to surgical treatment, one was quasi-experimental (Reese et al., 1996); eight were descriptive (Baker, 1992; Dropkin, 1997; Dropkin et al., 1983; Dropkin & Scott, 1983; Kagan et al., 2002; Langius et al., 1993; Lennie et al., 2001; Lockhart, 2000); and one was qualitative (Fritz, 2001). Of the

studies primarily related to patients undergoing RT, one was intervention testing (Walizer & Ephraim, 1996); one was a pilot clinical trial (Dodd et al., 2003); six were descriptive (Huang et al., 2000; Jaster, 1991; Meek et al., 2000; Ohrn & Sjoden, 2003; Rose-Ped et al., 2002; Shiba, 1997); and one was qualitative (Fritz). Only one study focused primarily on patients undergoing chemotherapy (Wilson, 1993).

Based on the results of these studies, specific eating difficulties have been identified that may occur prior to surgery and/or preoperative treatment. Mouth pain frequently accompanies these difficulties. Further description is needed on the clinical implications of preoperative eating difficulties and tolerance of treatment. Intervention studies designed to reduce mouth pain also are warranted. Instrumentation now is available to measure the relative severity of visible changes in appearance and self-presentation following surgical resection. Quantification of these concepts not only continues to facilitate further research but also validates the perceived impact on the patients as well as the nurses who care for them (Dropkin et al., 1983; Lockhart, 2000). A major gap remains in the literature, however, on the more comprehensive description and management of specific categories of disfigurement and dysfunction experienced by patients who have undergone head and neck surgery, particularly over time. As the result of several study findings, risk factors have been identified that increase length of hospitalization after head and neck cancer surgery (Dropkin, 1997; Kagan et al., 2002). It remains unclear, however, what measures are necessary to ameliorate this problem. Similarly, studies have identified many factors regarding complications of tube feedings (Reese et al., 1996). Although several suggestions are made for clinical intervention based on the results, these interventions must be empirically tested.

Patients' experiences of RT-induced mucositis and xerostomia have been clarified by the results of several studies (Dodd et al., 2003; Fritz, 2001; Huang et al., 2000; Ohrn & Sjoden, 2003; Rose-Ped et al., 2002; Shiba, 1997). Two studies tested interventions, but replication in larger samples is necessary before evidence-based changes in practice can occur. Although Rose-Ped et al. (2002) have suggested that tolerance of treatment may be related to the primary site, none of the studies that were reviewed, with the exception of Huang et al. (2000), who studied patients under treatment for nasopharyngeal cancer, used stratified sampling techniques accordingly.

Some controversy exists as to the occurrence and severity of pain and whether it is increased with swallowing. Perhaps this is contingent on the primary site or location of treatment ports as well, affecting various phases of the swallowing process. Again, stratification of samples may clarify this issue.

Interventions, such as the effectiveness of salt and soda to reduce mucositis (Dodd et al., 2003) and vegetable oil to reduce xerostomia (Walizer & Ephraim, 1996), not only are important findings in relation to enhancing patient comfort but also are practical and cost-effective solutions to critical problems for patients undergoing RT to the head and neck region. Numerous other phenomena, such as taste changes (Rose-Ped et al., 2002; Shiba, 1997), weight loss (Rose-Ped et al.; Shiba, 1997), skin changes (Huang et al., 2000), weakness, fatigue, and sleep disturbance (Meek et al., 2000; Rose-Ped et al.), need more accurate assessment and effective management, particularly in light of the extended time period required to administer RT but also in relation to long-term follow-up.

Patients' physical response to chemotherapy has not been well studied to date, perhaps because of the relatively small role this treatment modality has traditionally assumed in the treatment of head and neck cancer. With the use of increasingly rigorous treatment, including use of chemotherapy and its combination with RT, it is critical to note the findings of Huang et al. (2000) in that sequelae of RT may be exacerbated in those patients who have undergone prior chemotherapy. Additionally, an instrument now is available to measure the symptom experience and eating strategies specifically used by patients undergoing chemotherapy (Wilson, 1993).

Functional Recovery: Surgical Treatment

According to the Recovery Model (Scott & Eisendrath, 1986), functional recovery is conceptualized as adjustment in activities of daily living under the conditions of disease, treatment, and illness. Manifestations of this include extent of dependency on others for personal and social needs, as well as the social support system. The process of functional recovery includes reestablishment of activities of daily living, continuation of work activities with related feelings of usefulness, and reorganization of relationships with others (Scott & Eisendrath). Based on the literature reviewed, primary areas for study related to functional recovery in the surgical patient with head and neck cancer include social readjustment, quality of life, and feelings of usefulness.

Social Readjustment

One study conducted by Hancher (1988) was designed to explore how patients who have undergone total laryngectomy judge postoperative social adjustment and to identify difficulties encountered in resuming social roles. Social adjustment was defined as interaction after a critical life change within the social environment in occupational, marital, family, and community roles, plus the satisfaction associated with performance of these roles. The sample consisted of 19 total laryngectomees, 15 men and 4 women, with a mean age of 62 years. Time since surgery ranged from three months to nine years, with a mean of two years. A questionnaire designed to measure social adaptation was administered on two occasions in the form of an interview to detect changes in activity levels before and after surgery. The questionnaire included demographic data and questions related to areas of social adjust-

ment to work, leisure activities, interpersonal relations, and experience of negative public treatment. Overall, the majority of this sample judged postoperative social adjustment to be successful. Specifically, 38% of this sample was reemployed. This low figure is attributed to their being near retirement age. Minimal differences were reported, however, in resumption of social roles, such as family and social activities. Fifty-two percent of the sample experienced some negative public treatment but were not severely affected by it. Generally, those participants who cited a decrease in activities since surgery attributed it to aphonia and physical impairments.

Overall difficulty that may be experienced by the disfigured patient with head and neck cancer is illustrated by the results of a recent study on psychosocial rehabilitation after disfiguring injury or disease (Clarke & Cooper, 2001). This study was designed to identify the training needs of nurses working with disfigured patients. Although nurses have been identified as the healthcare professionals who may provide the most psychosocial support, less evidence shows that they feel confident in their ability to do so. A cross-sectional design of two groups of nurses working with either burn victims or disfigured patients with head and neck cancer were surveyed by questionnaire. Both groups rated their skills in psychosocial rehabilitation significantly lower than their skills in physical rehabilitation. Findings from this study indicated that healthcare professionals may themselves present barriers to the social readjustment of disfigured patients with head and neck cancer. Findings also implied that specific training and access to appropriate resources may facilitate nurses' ability to interact with this patient population.

More recently, the results of a qualitative study (Crighton, Goldberg, & Kagan, 2002) suggested the importance of the role of the nurse in enhancing feelings of usefulness in patients following their experience of head and neck cancer surgery. Seven patients participated in a study designed to develop an instrument. Content themes indicated that the interactive participation in this research project was both altruistic and beneficial for the individual participants. The research nurse played a particularly important role in the process of elucidating patients' relevant experiences. This likely was achieved through the nurse's ability to provide the participant with meaningful social contact in a safe and therapeutic context.

Quality of Life

Only one study was reviewed that directly examined the quality of life in patients with head and neck cancer (Reider, 1993). The purpose of the study was to determine if impairments such as speech understandability, normalcy of diet, and ability to eat in public were related to patients' perception of quality of life. The study also investigated possible relationships between symptom distress and quality of life. A convenience sample of 34 patients participated in this descriptive correlational study. Performance status and symptom distress were assessed in relation to current perception of quality of life. Reestablishment of a relatively normal diet, ability to eat in public, and understandability of speech were each significantly and positively related to quality of life.

Functional Recovery: Radiation Therapy

Based on the literature review for functional recovery and RT for head and neck cancer, the studies reviewed primarily focused on extent of dependency on others and quality-of-life issues.

Dependency on Others

One of the earlier studies regarding social support and self-care in relation to quality of life in patients receiving RT was conducted in Thailand (Hanucharurnkul, 1989). One purpose of this study was to examine the relationships among social support, self-care, and quality of life in patients receiving RT while selected demographic factors were statistically controlled—age, marital and socioeconomic status, living arrangement, and stage and site of disease. The second purpose included testing a theoretical model that postulated that quality of life was predicted jointly by the selected factors, social support, and self-care; self-care was predicted jointly by demographic factors and social support. A convenience sample of 112 adult patients with cervical and head and neck cancer receiving RT was obtained from outpatient clinics in three hospitals. Researchers assessed quality of life, self-care, and social support. Results of the study indicated positive relationships among self-care, social support, and quality of life. Socioeconomic status, site of cancer, and self-care were significant predictors for reported quality of life. Socioeconomic status and social support also were significant predictors of self-care, whereas stage and site of cancer seemed to predict self-care indirectly through social support. Factor analysis of the quality-of-life index used in this study yielded three meaningful factors: well-being, symptom control, and social concern.

Quality of Life

Rose and Yates (2001) explored the quality of life for 58 outpatients during and after a course of RT for head and neck cancer. Data were collected across three time (T) points: T1 (first week of treatment), T2 (last week of treatment), and T3 (one month after treatment). Patients completed two measures that assessed physical, emotional, functional, and social aspects of well-being. Repeated measures of multivariate analysis of variance and post hoc t-tests were performed to assess changes in quality of life over the three time points. Results indicated overall increased levels of physical and functional symptoms, head and neck–specific concerns, and depression

between T1 and T2. However, except for depression, some improvement occurred between scores on each of these measures of physical and functional well-being between T2 and T3, although this improvement did not reach pretreatment levels. The scales assessing social and emotional well-being showed no significant changes across time.

Functional Recovery: Chemotherapy

Quality of Life

One study reviewed on the relationship between oral health and quality of life included a cohort of patients with head and neck cancer undergoing RT and/or the second or third cycle of chemotherapy (Ohrn, Sjoden, Whalin, & Elf, 2001). Researchers administered a questionnaire to assess quality of life that included questions specific to the head and neck patient population at the beginning and end of treatment. Results indicated that quality of life tended to decrease over time, and oral symptoms increased. Patients who reported that their oral symptoms and lower quality of life had influenced their everyday life reported more severe oral symptoms and lower quality of life at the end of treatment, when the oral symptoms were most severe.

Summary: Functional Recovery

The research reviewed regarding patients' functional recovery following diagnosis and treatment of head and neck cancer consisted of descriptive studies. Two investigations examined the recovery process with regard to social readjustment after total laryngectomy (Hancher, 1988), as well as to specific problems with eating and speech articulation (Reider, 1993). The importance of the nurse's role in facilitating functional recovery also is beginning to emerge (Clarke & Cooper, 2001; Crighton et al., 2002). Quality of life was described in a sample of patients who had sustained postsurgical sensorimotor disabilities (Reider). Two studies examined quality-of-life issues in patients undergoing RT (Hanucharurnkul, 1989; Rose & Yates, 2001). One study examined the relationship between oral health and quality of life in patients undergoing RT and/or chemotherapy (Ohrn et al., 2001).

The results of these studies indicated that postoperative social adjustment indeed is possible over time in aphonic patients (Hancher, 1988). Those patients who sustain severe disfigurement, however, may receive less than adequate teaching and counseling in relation to psychosocial rehabilitation because of nurses' discomfort in confronting and interacting with disfigured patients (Clarke & Cooper, 2001). This finding is particularly alarming in light of Crighton et al.'s (2002) results, which indicated the critical role that nurses may assume in postoperative patients' functional recovery. Quality of life was negatively affected in the surgical patient population when sensorimotor deficits had been sustained (Reider, 1993). The findings indicated that as the impairment(s) improved, so did quality of life. The factor of adjustment over time also may be operational in this setting with body image reintegration.

In patients undergoing RT, dependency on others was a major concern (Hanucharurnkul, 1989). Perhaps this was an issue because of the protracted nature of the treatment and subsequent extended time of need for personal and social support from others. Quality of life similarly diminished for RT patients during the experience of symptomatology (Rose & Yates, 2001), which supported previous research for this group of patients. Although quality of life improved with physical recovery, feelings of depression in this sample persisted through the last follow-up, at one month after treatment was completed. Finally, for those patients undergoing RT and/or chemotherapy (Ohrn et al., 2001), quality of life varied according to oral health throughout the course of treatment.

Based on the results of these studies, the ability to accurately diagnose and manage patients' physical and emotional symptoms within this context is critical to improve and enhance overall functional recovery, particularly quality of life in the increasing number of survivors of head and neck cancer treatment.

Cognitive Recovery: Surgical Treatment

Cognitive recovery is conceptualized as the regulation of mental representation under conditions of disease, treatment, and illness. Manifestations of this include alterations in self-concept and body image, which are primarily accomplished through the use of problem-focused coping strategies (Scott & Eisendrath, 1986). According to the literature reviewed, primary areas for study related to cognitive recovery in the surgical patient with head and neck cancer include alterations in body image through the use of problem-focused coping strategies as well as the specific problem-focused coping strategy of information seeking.

Body Image Alteration and Reintegration

The results of several studies (Dropkin, 1994, 1997; Dropkin et al., 1983; Dropkin & Scott, 1983) over the course of two decades have demonstrated the process of body image alteration with subsequent reintegration of surgical changes into self following head and neck cancer surgery. In early studies, observable behaviors that theoretically manifested body image alteration were clinically observed and monitored. The researchers concluded that self-care and resocialization were the major problem-focused coping behaviors used during the early period after surgery, which represented manifestations of body image alteration. Furthermore, the time frame, or specific postoperative day on which coping behaviors occurred, significantly correlated to the degree of disfigurement and dysfunction sustained in surgery (Dropkin & Scott). Although it remains unclear whether degree of postoperative disfigurement and dysfunction predicts body image reintegration, or assimilation of the postoperative deficit(s) that is acceptable to the individual, the results of more recent studies support the notion that patients who sustain more severe surgical deficits experience greater difficulty with body image alteration and reintegration (Dropkin, 1994, 1997; Krouse, Krouse, & Fabian, 1989). Moreover, the results of one study (Dropkin, 1997) implied that coping with body image alteration and reintegration may be related to length of postoperative hospitalization. Specifically, preoperative coping effectiveness was significantly reduced by prior cancer treatment(s) such as RT or chemotherapy and the anticipation of disfiguring surgery. Preoperative coping strategies were significantly and positively related to postoperative coping behaviors. Furthermore, it was concluded that wound healing clearly influenced both postoperative coping and length of postoperative hospital stay. Overall, body image reintegration was characterized by self-care, resocialization, and reduced anxiety levels (Dropkin, 1994, 1997).

Information Seeking

In a study designed specifically to describe common themes in the experiences and expressed informational needs of patients who have had head and neck cancer surgery, Newell, Ziegler, Stafford, and Lewin (2004) used semistructured qualitative interviews with 29 participants and 12 relatives or close friends present at the time of consultation with the surgeon. The focus of the interview schedule was the patients' and relatives' experiences of how the discussion was conducted, with particular reference to their perception of the amount and relevance of information they had been given; their ability to comprehend the information and its consequences; and the amount of choice they perceived that they had in the decision to undergo surgery. Several interesting conclusions resulted. Frequently, the initial discussion was conducted in the presence of several professionals, making it difficult for the patient and relative to focus on what was being said and inhibiting them from asking questions. Findings suggested that patients' information needs vary greatly, although not necessarily according to the type of surgery they are anticipating. Participants reported feeling unprepared for the long-term changes that occurred, particularly changes in lifestyle, including loss of employment and social life. Furthermore, they felt that informational support for up to six months after surgery was inadequate. The use of medical jargon and technical words frequently made comprehension difficult for patients. The majority of participants did not ask any questions nor perceive that there was a choice other than that recommended by the surgeon;

only three participants felt they had taken a proactive role in the decision-making process. Individuals who wanted to take an active role in the decision-making process reported difficulty in accessing the appropriate information. Finally, satisfaction with the information provided appeared to be primarily related to patients' ability to influence the course of the discussion such that their needs were met. According to consistency noted in participants' views, researchers concluded that information should be given in a quiet and private environment where patients did not feel rushed. All patients reported that they wanted information provided in simple language, and most wanted written information and diagrams as well. Overall, these findings demonstrated the need for the provision of individualized information.

Cognitive Recovery: Radiation Therapy

According to the literature reviewed on cognitive recovery and RT for head and neck cancer, the primary areas for study included information-seeking and patients' perception of the experience.

Information Seeking

Shieh, Wang, Tsai, and Tseng (1997) conducted a randomized clinical trial to compare the effect of three oral care protocols in delaying the onset of stomatitis and reducing oral injury in a sample of 30 patients undergoing RT for nasopharyngeal cancer. Participants were randomly assigned to one of three groups: those who received instructions on oral care at one day and one week before beginning RT, respectively, and the control group who received no specific instructions. According to oral assessment, researchers concluded that those patients who received information one week prior to the initiation of RT experienced later onset of stomatitis than those in either of the two other groups. Similarly, they experienced a lesser degree of oral injury. It was concluded that giving information about mouth care one week prior to RT was most effective in delaying the onset of stomatitis and reducing oral injury in patients with nasopharyngeal cancer. These findings supported earlier research (Grant, 1987) on the effects of a structured teaching program for patients with cancer undergoing head and neck RT on anorexia, nutritional status, functional status, treatment response, and quality of life. The study sample consisted of 41 participants who were randomized to the structured teaching program (n = 21) or the "usual care" group (n = 20). Results showed significantly higher scores on nutritional knowledge for the experimental group at the end of the treatment period. Although additional statistical significance was not achieved, the findings suggested that a structured teaching program may reduce decreased dietary intake during RT despite decreased appetite in the patient with head and neck cancer.

Perception of the Experience

Stajduhar et al. (2000) conducted a qualitative study to enhance understanding of the experience as well as the educational needs of patients receiving iodine-131 for the treatment of thyroid cancer. The sample consisted of 5 men and 22 women who had received iodine-131 within the previous two years. Four major themes emerged from the analysis: (a) recognizing the totality of the cancer experience, or how patients perceived their cancer experience, (b) being isolated, both socially and physically, (c) recognizing the totality of the treatment experience, both pre- and post-treatment, and (d) understanding barriers to treatment, such as frustration associated with treatment delays. The researchers concluded that healthcare workers require a better understanding of thyroid disease, its treatment, and side effects. Moreover, specific educational programs for staff as well as patients were recommended to adequately address the comprehensive care of this patient population.

Cognitive Recovery: Chemotherapy

One study was reviewed on cognitive recovery from chemotherapy treatment for head and neck cancer. In a study designed to describe the perception of education, self-rated knowledge, and attitudes toward oral care among nurses who care for patients with head and neck cancer (among other patient populations with cancer), a total of 18% felt uncomfortable in discussing oral hygiene with the patients, and 45% objected to examining the oral cavity (Ohrn, 2000). This finding supported Newell et al.'s (2004) results, in that healthcare professionals may themselves present barriers to patients' cognitive recovery or ability to obtain adequate information regarding their condition.

Summary: Cognitive Recovery

Several interesting findings are available based on the research concerning the cognitive dimension of recovery from head and neck cancer treatment. Self-care and resocialization were identified as observable and measurable behaviors used by postsurgical patients to cope with the body image alterations of disfigurement and dysfunction (Dropkin & Scott, 1983). Ultimately, body image integration represents maximal reemergence of the premorbid individual as the individual adapts the mental representation of presurgical appearance and function to postsurgical reality. The results of three studies confirmed that patients undergoing head and neck cancer surgery who have increased levels of facial disfigurement and sensorimotor dysfunction experience increasing difficulty coping with the process of body image reintegration (Dropkin, 1994; Dropkin & Scott, 1983; Krouse et al.,

1989). Similarly, coping behavior is adversely affected by presurgical RT or chemotherapy, anticipation of disfigurative surgery, ineffective presurgical coping strategies, and wound healing complications. Alternatively, individuals with effective strategies for coping prior to surgery demonstrated increased coping behaviors after surgery (Dropkin, 1997).

More recently, Newell et al. (2004) have clearly documented information-seeking behavior, an effective problem-focused coping strategy, in the presurgical head and neck population. Major barriers to patients' utilization of this coping strategy, however, often are presented by healthcare professionals themselves.

In patients undergoing RT to the head and neck area, information-seeking, with the ultimate outcome of increased knowledge (Grant, 1987), has been shown to be effective in delaying the onset of mucositis and reducing the degree of stomatitis (Shieh et al., 1997). In a qualitative study, patients undergoing radioactive iodine-131 treatment for thyroid cancer specifically requested more information about their disease to facilitate coping (Stajduhar et al., 2000).

Finally, those patients undergoing chemotherapy similarly may have difficulty obtaining information regarding oral care because nurses may be reluctant to discuss such issues with them (Ohrn, 2000).

Emotional Recovery: Surgical Treatment

Emotional recovery denotes expression of the feelings generated by changes in mental representation. The meaning of the disease, treatment, and illness predicts the emotional response. The process of emotional recovery includes intra-psychic regulation designed to reduce psychological distress (Scott & Eisendrath, 1986). Studies reviewed concerning emotional recovery with surgical treatment focused on patients' experience of anxiety and depression.

Anxiety

In a prospective study designed to investigate the relationship of anxiety and the use of problem-focused coping strategies to self-care and resocialization in patients who sustain facial disfigurement/dysfunction, Dropkin (1994) identified several sources of anxiety for this population during the preoperative and early postoperative period. The sample consisted of 75 adults who were about to sustain moderate to severe disfigurement/dysfunction associated with head and neck cancer surgery. Preoperative anticipation of disfigurative surgery was associated with extremely high levels of anxiety, and overall coping effectiveness was diminished in this sample. Furthermore, preoperative anxiety negatively correlated with age and positively correlated with postoperative anxiety. Coping behavior, or total self-care, significantly and negatively correlated to anxiety on postoperative days 4 and 5. For the three

days under study, however, the relationship between self-care and anxiety became stronger, indicating that performance of self-care on postoperative day 4 was related to reduced anxiety on postoperative day 5. In other words, self-care appeared to precede reduction in anxiety in this sample.

Depression

In Fritz's (2001) pilot qualitative study of three patients who had undergone head and neck surgery, depression emerged as a major concern. The two male patients appeared to have a more positive outlook on their subsequent quality of life; the female patient, however, openly admitted her feelings of depression. Several antidepressants prescribed by a psychiatrist only exacerbated mouth dryness in this patient, and she refused further psychotropic medication. She also complained of insomnia. And although she performed volunteer work, she continued to experience feelings of worthlessness. Fritz concluded that the patients in this sample experienced a myriad of emotional distress, including feelings of guilt, anxiety, and helplessness, in addition to depression.

Emotional Recovery: Radiation Therapy

The literature reviewed on emotional recovery and RT revealed two primary aspects of emotional distress: loss of self and depression.

Loss of Self

The phrase "loss of self" ultimately refers to loss of self-in-tegrity and was one of the major themes that emerged in Wells' (1998) qualitative study concerning the impact of RT on patients after completion of treatment. Generally, emotional recovery was noted to be less rapid than physical recovery. Some patients in this sample of 12 were left with residual functional problems related to combined surgery and RT, such as salivary drooling or speech impairment, that continued to be a source of emotional distress long after completion of treatment. Moreover, many patients experienced great apprehension about resuming work, hobbies, and relationships with others. Patients experienced an apparent loss of confidence as well as self-worth, possibly exacerbated by the visible effects of treatment. Many patients appeared to experience social anxiety (i.e., reluctance to be seen by others). Often, confidence seemed to reemerge only with improvement in symptoms or the ability to function normally again. Subsequently, the patients may have regained some of their self-integrity.

Depression

In support of Wells' (1998) findings, Rose and Yates (2001) determined increased levels of depression between T1 and T2 that persisted between T2 and T3 despite some improvement in physical symptomatology and functional well-being.

More recently, in a study of patients who had undergone nasopharyngeal RT (Lai et al., 2003), researchers concluded that although overall symptom distress was mild to moderate in patients who had previously completed RT (n = 44, less than one year; n = 38, less than three years), those subjects actively undergoing treatment (n = 33) reported a myriad of moderately distressful symptoms. Regression analysis revealed that catastrophic thinking, associated with symptom distress, predicted significantly lower levels of hope across the total sample. Nursing interventions to reduce negative thinking and enhance hope are suggested based on study results.

Emotional Recovery: Chemotherapy

No studies were reviewed that addressed emotional recovery and chemotherapy for patients with head and neck cancer.

Summary: Emotional Recovery

Several studies have described the devastating and persistent emotional responses to treatment for head and neck cancer. Extremely high levels of anxiety have been documented with anticipation of disfigurative surgery. Similarly, high levels of anxiety tended to occur in younger patients and were adversely associated with subsequent coping efforts after surgery (Dropkin, 1997). Of major clinical significance is that performance of self-care significantly reduced anxiety by the fifth postoperative day (Dropkin, 1997). This finding cannot be generalized, however, beyond the study sample, and further study, such as replication, is warranted.

Depression also has been described in patients undergoing surgery and/or RT (Fritz, 2001). Emotional recovery, in general, required more time in patients who had undergone surgery as well as RT according to Wells' (1998) findings. Loss of self-integrity and self-confidence with increased feelings of apprehension about resuming work and relationships also occurred (Wells). Depression may persist despite improvement in physical and functional dimensions of recovery. Similarly, catastrophizing, a negative cognition, requires ongoing assessment long after treatment has been discontinued.

No studies were reviewed on emotional recovery in patients receiving chemotherapy for head and neck cancer.

Future Directions

During the past 25 years, a growing body of research has developed that is beginning to improve the lives of those who have been affected by cancer of the head and neck. According to this review, however, several gaps exist in the literature that need to be addressed. The majority of the studies reviewed are plagued by small sample sizes. Although many factors determine the sample size that is appropriate for a quantitative study, sample size is a major consideration in the validity of a study as well as generalizability of study results. This problem is pervasive in nursing research in that external funding sources increasingly are requiring that the researcher predetermine the exact sample size needed for a study; subsequently, power analysis is being used more frequently (Nieswiadomy, 2002). The patient population with head and neck cancer is relatively small; consequently, it may be particularly difficult to obtain sufficiently large samples for study. One solution, as suggested by Nieswiadomy, is replication of studies, thereby exponentially increasing sample sizes. Another possible solution might be the formation of regional or national head and neck cancer nursing research networks so that one study sample may originate from several sites.

The overwhelming majority of the studies reviewed were descriptive in nature. With increased sample sizes and/or increased research designed in a systematic fashion to enhance the body of scientific knowledge, intervention-testing or experimental studies need to be conducted to facilitate evidence-based practice for this patient population.

Increasing stratification of study samples is important in ensuring clarity and accuracy of study outcomes. Additionally, more qualitative studies would greatly enhance the understanding of the experience of diagnosis and treatment of head and neck cancer. Quantitative instrumentation may not consistently measure the unique problems of this patient population. The majority of the studies reviewed were of a cross-sectional design. A significant gap exists in the literature, however, regarding the manner in which patients' recovery occurs and changes over time. More studies with a longitudinal design are needed. It especially is critical for this patient population because with increasingly rigorous medical therapy, including combinations of treatment modalities, patients are living longer with the sequelae of treatment.

Finally, several topics urgently need to be addressed in this patient population that have not been empirically studied to date. These include sexuality issues; ethnicity issues, including studies of poor and underserved populations; and how nurses may play a role in early prevention and detection (Powe & Finnie, 2004). End-of-life issues for patients with head and neck cancer are similarly important for study, and pain related to all treatment modalities continues to be a research priority (Cohen, Harle, Woll, Despa, & Munsell, 2004). Nurses need to understand the true impact that the diagnosis and treatment of head and neck cancer have on patients' lives to administer the most comprehensive, compassionate, and accurate care based on nursing science. Although patients with head and neck cancer constitute only a small percentage of all patient populations with cancer, their unique and emergent needs provide compelling nursing phenomena for scientific study with subsequent effective intervention and predictable outcomes.

References

Baker, C. (1992). Factors associated with rehabilitation in head and neck cancer. *Cancer Nursing, 15,* 395–400.

Clarke, A., & Cooper, C. (2001). Psychosocial rehabilitation after disfiguring injury or disease: Investigating the training needs of specialist nurses. *Journal of Advanced Nursing, 34,* 18–26.

Crighton, M.H., Goldberg, A.N., & Kagan, S.H. (2002). Reciprocity for patients with head and neck cancer participating in an instrument development project. *Oncology Nursing Forum, 29,* E127–E131.

Cohen, M.Z., Harle, M., Woll, A.M., Despa, S., & Munsell, M.F. (2004). Delphi survey of nursing research priorities. *Oncology Nursing Forum, 31,* 1011–1018.

Dodd, M.J., Miaskowski, C., Greenspan, D., MacPhail, L., Shih, A.S., Shiba, G., et al. (2003). Radiation-induced mucositis: A randomized clinical trial of micronized sucralfate versus salt and soda mouthwashes. *Cancer Investigation, 21*(1), 21–33.

Dropkin, M.J. (1994). *Anxiety, problem-focused coping strategies, disfigurement/dysfunction and postoperative coping behaviors associated with head and neck cancer.* Unpublished doctoral dissertation, New York University, New York.

Dropkin, M.J. (1997). Coping with disfigurement/dysfunction and length of hospital stay after head and neck cancer surgery. *ORL—Head and Neck Nursing, 15*(1), 22–26.

Dropkin, M.J., Malgady, R.G., Scott, D.W., Oberst, M.T., & Strong, E.W. (1983). Scaling of disfigurement and dysfunction in postoperative head and neck patients. *Head and Neck Surgery, 6,* 559–570.

Dropkin, M.J., & Scott, D.W. (1983). Body image reintegration and coping effectiveness after head and neck surgery. *The Journal (Official Publication of the Society of Otorhinolaryngology and Head-Neck Nurses), 2*(1), 7–16.

Fritz, D.J. (2001). Life experiences of head and neck cancer survivors: A pilot study. *ORL—Head and Neck Nursing, 19*(4), 9–13.

Grant, M.M. (1987). Effects of a structured teaching program for cancer patients undergoing head and neck radiation therapy on anorexia, nutritional status, functional status, treatment response and quality of life. *Dissertation Abstracts International, 48*(11B), 3248.

Hancher, K. (1988). Social adjustment of laryngectomy patients. *The Journal (Official Publication of the Society of Otorhinolaryngology and Head-Neck Nurses), 6*(2), 4–8.

Hanucharurnkul, S. (1989). Predictors of self-care in cancer patients receiving radiotherapy. *Cancer Nursing, 12,* 21–27.

Huang, H., Wilkie, D.J., Schubert, M.M., & Ting, L. (2000). Symptom profile of nasopharyngeal cancer patients during radiation therapy. *Cancer Practice, 8,* 274–281.

Jaster, S.E. (1991). Self-care burden with radiotherapy for head and neck cancer. *Masters Abstracts International, 30*(1), 95.

Kagan, S.H., Chalian, A.A., Goldberg, A.N., Rontal, M.L., Weinstein, G.S., Prior, B., et al. (2002). Impact of age on clinical care pathway length of stay following complex head and neck resection. *Head and Neck, 24,* 545–548.

Krouse, J.H., Krouse, H.J., & Fabian, R.L. (1989). Adaptation to surgery for head and neck cancer. *Laryngoscope, 99,* 789–794.

Lai, Y.H., Chang, J.T., Keefe, F.J., Chiou, C.F., Chen, S.C., Feng, S.C., et al. (2003). Symptom distress, catastrophic thinking, and hope in nasopharyngeal carcinoma patients. *Cancer Nursing, 26,* 485–493.

Langius, A., Bjorvell, H., & Lind, M.G. (1993). Oral- and pharyngeal-cancer patients' perceived symptoms and health. *Cancer Nursing, 16,* 214–221.

Lennie, T.A., Christman, S.K., & Jadack, R.A. (2001). Educational needs and altered eating habits following a total laryngectomy. *Oncology Nursing Forum. 28,* 667–674.

Lockhart, J. (2000). Nurses' perceptions of head and neck oncology patients after surgery: Severity of facial disfigurement and patient gender. *Plastic Surgical Nursing, 20*(2), 68–80.

Meek, P.M., Nail, L.M., Barsevick, A., Schwartz, A.L., Stephen, S., Whitmer, K., et al. (2000). Psychometric testing of fatigue instruments for use with cancer patients. *Nursing Research, 49,* 181–190.

Newell, R., Ziegler, L., Stafford, N., & Lewin, R. (2004). The information needs of head and neck cancer patients prior to surgery. *Annals of The Royal College of Surgeons of England, 86,* 407–410.

Nieswiadomy, R.M. (2002). *Foundations of nursing research* (4th ed.). Upper Saddle River, NJ: Prentice Hall.

Ohrn, K.E. (2000). Oral care in cancer nursing. *European Journal of Cancer Care, 9,* 22–29.

Ohrn, K.E., & Sjoden, P.O. (2003). Experiences of oral care inpatients with haematological malignancies or head and neck cancer. *European Journal of Cancer Care, 12,* 274–282.

Ohrn, K.E., Sjoden, P.O., Whalin, Y.B., & Elf, M. (2001). Oral health and quality of life among patients with head and neck cancer or haematological malignancies. *Supportive Care in Cancer, 9,* 528–538.

Oncology Nursing Society. (2004). *Cancer research and cancer clinical trials.* Retrieved January 7, 2005, from http://www.ons.org/publications/positions/CancerResearch.shtml

Powe, B.D., & Finnie, R. (2004). Knowledge of oral cancer risk factors among African Americans: Do nurses have a role? *Oncology Nursing Forum, 31,* 785–791.

Reese, J.L., Means, M.E., Hanrahan, K., Clearman, B., Colwill, M., & Dawson, C. (1996). Diarrhea associated with nasogastric feedings. *Oncology Nursing Forum, 23,* 59–68.

Reider, K.S. (1993). Quality of life in the patient with head and neck cancer. *Masters Abstracts International, 32*(2), 600.

Rose, P., & Yates, P. (2001). Quality of life experienced by patients receiving radiation treatment for cancers of the head and neck. *Cancer Nursing, 24,* 255–263.

Rose-Ped, A.M., Bellm, L.A., Epstein, J.B., Trotti, A., Gwede, C., & Fuchs, H. (2002). Complications of radiation therapy for head and neck cancers: The patient's perspective. *Cancer Nursing, 25,* 461–467.

Scott, D.W., & Eisendrath, S.J. (1986). Dynamics of the recovery process following initial diagnosis of breast cancer. *Journal of Psychosocial Oncology, 3,* 53–66.

Scott, D.W., Oberst, M.T., & Dropkin, M.J. (1980). A stress-coping model. *Advances in Nursing Science, 3*(1), 9–23.

Shiba, G.H. (1997). Radiation therapy-related mucositis, mucositis pain, and self-care behaviors of the head and neck cancer patient. *Dissertation Abstracts International, 58*(8B), 4147.

Shieh, S.H., Wang, S.T., Tsai, S.T., & Tseng, C.C. (1997). Mouth care for nasopharyngeal cancer patients undergoing radiotherapy. *Oral Oncology, 33,* 36–41.

Stajduhar, K.I., Neithercut, J., Chu, E., Pham, P., Rohde, J., Sicotte, A., et al. (2000). Thyroid cancer: Patients' experiences of receiving iodine-131 therapy. *Oncology Nursing Forum, 27,* 1213–1218.

Walizer, E.M., & Ephraim, P.A. (1996). Double-blind cross-over controlled clinical trial of vegetable oil versus Xerolube for xerostomia: An expanded study abstract. *ORL—Head and Neck Nursing, 14*(1), 11–12.

Wells, M. (1998). The hidden experience of radiotherapy to the head and neck: A qualitative study of patients after completion of treatment. *Journal of Advanced Nursing, 28,* 840–848.

Wilson, P.R. (1993). Symptoms and eating during cancer treatment (chemotherapy). *Dissertation Abstracts International, 54*(4B), 1897.

Index

The letter f *following a page number indicates that relevant content appears in a figure; the letter* t, *in a table.*